Winning Health Promotion Strategies

Anne Marie Ludovici-Connolly, MS, CHFS

Hewitt Associates
University of Rhode Island

Human Kinetics

Library of Congress Cataloging-in-Publication Data

Ludovici-Connolly, Anne Marie, 1959-
    Winning health promotion strategies / Anne Marie Ludovici-Connolly.
        p. ; cm.
    Includes bibliographical references and index.
    ISBN-13: 978-0-7360-7965-5 (soft cover)
    ISBN-10: 0-7360-7965-3 (soft cover)
    1. Employee health promotion. I. Title.
    [DNLM: 1. Health Promotion--methods. 2. Health Promotion--organization & administration.
3. Program Development. WA 590 L943 2010]
    RC969.H43L83 2010
    362.1068'3--dc22

                                2009046275

ISBN-10: 0-7360-7965-3 (print)
ISBN-13: 978-0-7360-7965-5 (print)

The Web addresses cited in this text were current as of January 21, 2010, unless otherwise noted.

Acquisitions Editor: Myles Schrag; **Developmental Editor:** Amanda S. Ewing; **Assistant Editor:** Casey A. Gentis; **Copyeditor:** Patsy Fortney; **Indexer:** Andrea Hepner; **Permission Manager:** Dalene Reeder; **Graphic Designer:** Nancy Rasmus; **Graphic Artist:** Yvonne Griffith; **Cover Designer:** Keith Blomberg; **Photographer (cover):** Fancy/Veer/age fotostock; **Art Manager:** Kelly Hendren; **Associate Art Manager:** Alan L. Wilborn; **Illustrator:** Alan L. Wilborn; **Printer:** Versa Press

Printed in the United States of America   10 9 8 7 6 5 4 3 2 1

The paper in this book is certified under a sustainable forestry program.

Human Kinetics
Web site: www.HumanKinetics.com

United States: Human Kinetics
P.O. Box 5076
Champaign, IL 61825-5076
800-747-4457
e-mail: humank@hkusa.com

Canada: Human Kinetics
475 Devonshire Road Unit 100
Windsor, ON N8Y 2L5
800-465-7301 (in Canada only)
e-mail: info@hkcanada.com

Europe: Human Kinetics
107 Bradford Road
Stanningley
Leeds LS28 6AT, United Kingdom
+44 (0) 113 255 5665
e-mail: hk@hkeurope.com

Australia: Human Kinetics
57A Price Avenue
Lower Mitcham, South Australia 5062
08 8372 0999
e-mail: info@hkaustralia.com

New Zealand: Human Kinetics
P.O. Box 80
Torrens Park, South Australia 5062
0800 222 062
e-mail: info@hknewzealand.com

E4695

This book is dedicated to the loving memory of Bernardino Nicandro Ludovici, Jr., and Bernardino Nicandro Ludovici, Sr.

Bernardino Nicandro Ludovici, Jr., my dear, beloved late brother Dino, left us much too soon but was, and will always be, a shining star in our lives. Dino's life continually inspires me, and many other people whose lives he touched, to think beyond ourselves and to continually and consistently strive to be kind and compassionate.

Bernardino Nicandro Ludovici, Sr., my beloved late daddy, "Benny Gooch," who I will always love and remember for teaching me so many things about what's most important in life: love and gratitude. He also taught me that anything is possible if you pursue your dreams with dedication, passion, and perseverance.

CONTENTS

ACTIVITY FINDER   vii

FOREWORD   xi

PREFACE   xiii

ACKNOWLEDGMENTS   xxi

PART I   Understanding Wellness Initiatives   1

1   Making Wellness Work in Various Settings   3

Are you a wellness professional looking for different markets in which to offer your services? Do you know all of the settings offering wellness programs today? This chapter addresses national initiatives such as the National Physical Activity Plan, the U.S. Department of Health and Human Services Physical Activity Guidelines, and the First Lady's *Let's Move* campaign. The chapter also addresses the National Governors Association Healthy America call to action: wellness where we live, work, and learn. Learn how these calls to action can involve you!

2   Developing Successful Wellness Initiatives   15

Have you observed or read about an organization that is offering an excellent wellness initiative and wondered how it got there? Or, have you thought, Where do I begin? If so, this chapter is for you! Step-by-step guidelines help you develop a best-in-class wellness program. Read this chapter and next year we could be reading about you!

3   Creating Engaging Wellness Initiatives   43

Have the usual suspects been showing up at your wellness programs? If you are looking to engage different participants, retain the same, and draw in more, this chapter is for you! This chapter reveals several innovative techniques and strategies and outlines several ways to engage new, as well as more, people in your programs. This chapter will help you think outside of the box to pump up your participation rates.

4   Improving and Expanding Existing Wellness Initiatives   69

Are you looking to take your existing wellness program to the next level? Have you been looking for ways to evaluate or benchmark your existing program? This chapter provides a variety of ideas, tools, and resources to assist you in kicking it up a notch!

PART II   Winning Wellness Programs   81

5   Physical Activity Programs   83

If you are looking for physical activity programs to engage new, as well as more participants, consider offering programs that are shorter-duration, social, and fun. The programs in this chapter will get people out of their chairs and moving!

6   Nutrition Programs   105

Tired of the same old nutrition education programs? The programs in this chapter will inspire even junk-food lovers to attend!

7   General Health and Prevention Programs   123

Are you looking for creative programs that not only educate but also motivate participants? This chapter provides a variety of programs that range from reminders and motivating e-mails to full-scale behavior change interventions.

REFERENCES   170
INDEX   172
ABOUT THE AUTHOR   177

ACTIVITY FINDER

This activity finder will help you locate programs that fit your specific needs. You can select programs based on a variety of criteria:

- Setting (community, worksite, or school)
- Cost (low, medium, or high)
- Type (awareness, intervention, or education)
- Topic (physical activity, nutrition, or general health and prevention)

Page numbers are listed for all of the activities, too, so that you can easily turn to the program you want to implement.

Icon Key

Community =

Worksite =

School =

Low = (under $100)

Medium = ($100- $1,000)

High = (greater than $1,000)

Awareness =

Intervention =

Education =

Physical activity =

Nutrition =

General health and pre-vention =

Program	Page number	SETTING		COST			TYPE			TOPIC		
		(community/globe)	(school bus/radio)	$	$$	$$$$	(screening/eye)	(policy/cycle)	(education/grad cap)	(physical activity)	(nutrition/organs)	(heart health)
10-10-10	88	✓	✓	✓			✓					
15 for 15	124	✓	✓	✓				✓	✓	✓		✓
ABC for Fitness	90	✓	✓	✓				✓		✓		
Active Living Every Day	84	✓	✓	✓	✓			✓	✓	✓		
All You Can Eat	119	✓	✓	✓					✓		✓	
ALwell Incentives	155	✓	✓	✓	✓	✓		✓				✓
An Apple a Day	114	✓	✓	✓	✓			✓			✓	
Breast Health for Seniors	134	✓		✓	✓	✓		✓				✓
Colossal Colon	138	✓				✓		✓				✓
Community Cookbook	115	✓	✓	✓	✓	✓			✓		✓	
DelaWELL University	165	✓	✓	✓	✓	✓		✓	✓			✓
Drink Up	112	✓	✓	✓				✓			✓	
Farmers Markets	109	✓	✓	✓				✓	✓		✓	
Fitness Bee	102	✓	✓	✓				✓	✓	✓	✓	
Fitting in Fitness	91	✓	✓				✓	✓	✓	✓		
Healthy Book Club	164	✓	✓	✓					✓			✓
Healthy Eating Every Day	121	✓	✓	✓	✓			✓			✓	
Healthy Meetings	116	✓	✓	✓	✓			✓			✓	

Program	Page number	SETTING		COST			TYPE			TOPIC		
				$	$$	$$$						
Join the Club	101	✓	✓	✓			✓		✓	✓		
Just Move It	97	✓	✓	✓				✓	✓	✓		
Kick Colds and Flu	132	✓	✓	✓			✓		✓			✓
Know Your Health	157	✓	✓	✓				✓				✓
Know Your Numbers	148	✓	✓	✓	✓			✓				✓
Lactation Support	151	✓	✓	✓	✓		✓	✓				✓
Laugh It Up!	125	✓	✓	✓	✓		✓	✓				✓
Let's Dance	104	✓	✓	✓	✓			✓		✓		
Lunch and Learn	110	✓	✓	✓	✓		✓	✓	✓		✓	
Make It Stick	144	✓	✓	✓			✓	✓		✓		✓
Moving Meetings	96	✓	✓	✓		✓	✓	✓		✓		
Musical Happy Hour	130	✓	✓	✓			✓	✓				✓
My Pledge	159	✓	✓	✓			✓	✓				✓
Nutrition Detectives	106	✓	✓	✓				✓	✓		✓	
Observe Health	150	✓	✓	✓		✓	✓		✓			✓
PawSox and Prostates	135	✓		✓		✓	✓	✓				✓
Pet Therapy	131	✓	✓	✓			✓	✓				✓
Pink Spirit Week	140	✓	✓	✓			✓	✓	✓			✓
Play Ball	95	✓	✓	✓				✓		✓		
Portion Distortion	108	✓	✓	✓				✓	✓		✓	
Pro-Change	141	✓	✓	✓		✓	✓		✓			✓

>> continued

Program	Page number	SETTING (community)	SETTING (media/school)	COST $	COST $$	COST $$$	TYPE (eye)	TYPE (arrow)	TYPE (grad cap)	TOPIC (active)	TOPIC (glasses)	TOPIC (heart)
Raytheon Healthy Worksite Award	153	✓	✓	✓				✓				✓
School Health Index	142		✓	✓				✓				✓
Screen Savers	168	✓	✓	✓			✓					✓
Shape Up the Nation	93		✓	✓	✓		✓	✓		✓		
SparkPeople	100	✓	✓	✓				✓		✓		
StairWELL to Better Health	86	✓	✓	✓	✓		✓			✓		
Stop, Stretch, and Breathe	126	✓	✓	✓				✓				✓
Stress-Less Day	128	✓	✓	✓	✓		✓		✓			✓
Sun Smarts	137	✓		✓	✓	✓	✓	✓				✓
TrestleTree Health Coaching	169	✓	✓	✓	✓	✓	✓	✓				✓
Veggin' Out	122	✓	✓	✓	✓		✓		✓		✓	
Virtual Reminders	161	✓	✓	✓			✓					✓
Vitality	162	✓	✓	✓	✓			✓				✓
Wellness Impact Scorecard	154	✓		✓	✓			✓				
WIIFM: What's in It For Me?	118	✓	✓	✓			✓		✓		✓	✓
YMCA's Healthy Family Home	146	✓	✓	✓			✓		✓			✓

The notion of wellness is rapidly evolving. Fitness supplies are readily available, as are weight-loss programs. Workout gyms are everywhere, including in many office buildings. Flu shots and other prevention strategies are increasing in prevalence. And yet, against this backdrop, we continue to wrestle with societal issues such as obesity, poor eating habits, and physical inactivity. As a result, we see increases in the rates of diabetes, heart disease, and cancer.

The challenge with wellness, it seems, is getting people started and keeping them on track. That is what this book is about.

For the past year, I have had the pleasure of working with, and learning from, Anne Marie (Annie) Ludovici. As Annie notes in the book, she has been called a wellness rock star, and that is precisely why we hired her to join us at Hewitt Associates. Hewitt is a global human resources services firm, consulting with companies to design and implement and communicate a wide range of human resources, retirement, investment management, health management, compensation, and talent management strategies. I lead Hewitt's health management consulting business, and in that capacity work with employers to help them solve the vexing challenge of inspiring the people in their workforce to change their behaviors against a backdrop of rising health care costs, declining individual health, and increasing employee absence.

Our employer clients continue to tell us, regardless of external economic conditions, that employee health is a critical issue. In February 2009, we issued a survey report, *Challenges for Health Care in Uncertain Times*, in which we shared that employers rated keeping employees healthy as their most critical workforce issue. Moreover, those same employers told us that keeping employees healthy to improve productivity was the second most critical *business* issue, after managing cost. One year later, despite continued economic challenges, employers continued to rank improvement of employee health as a top workforce and business issue. Employers get that a healthy, present, and productive workforce drives business success.

At Hewitt, we believe that employers need to move beyond the short-term focus on cost management to strategically engage in helping those who are healthy stay that way, and in helping those who are ill to get better and to live more successfully with their conditions. We challenge our clients to move beyond just thinking about health care to a more fundamental role in driving improved health for their employees and their family members.

We believe that we need to walk that walk ourselves. For our associates at Hewitt, we've launched a program we call Choose Health, with online support information, live coaching, and on-site services in our major locations, as well as incentives for important activities such as completing a health risk questionnaire with biometric data. Recently, we launched a 12-week pilot program for our health management consultants through Shape Up the Nation, a social networking program (see chapter 5). The results were incredible: In a group of fewer than 350 people, we lost nearly 1,000 pounds

(454 kg), walked more than 128 million miles (206 million km), and created a sense of excitement and buzz that continued months after the official end of the program.

For me personally, our program was a great motivator. Every day, when I get home from work, my kids ask me how many steps I took that day (my answer usually is followed by something along the lines of, "Daddy! That's not enough steps!"). My personal wellness journey has become a family journey. My wife, Kerstin, wears a pedometer like mine, and our sons Matthew and Ryan ask how many steps we each have as they play basketball, soccer, and baseball. Where we are now has evolved from where we began with my successful venture into Weight Watchers, during which my then-six-year-old learned math by counting points with me.

For many employers, and for many health care professionals—in fact, for anyone who reads this book—the idea of launching a behavior-changing, fun, and engaging wellness strategy may seem impossible. This book is all about helping you. It does not just underscore the importance of wellness; it actually gives you very real examples of how to make it work.

I wish you much success, and good health, as you read this book and put its messages to work for you.

Jim Winkler

U.S. Health Management Practice Leader, Hewitt

Winning Health Promotion Strategies is a resource guide for professionals working in worksite, community, and school settings. Anyone interested in launching or improving existing wellness initiatives or programs will benefit from this book.

Winning Health Promotion Strategies is a "cookbook" that provides detailed information on successful wellness strategies in the form of comprehensive wellness initiatives as well as individual wellness programs. It features recipes for programs that focus on awareness, education, and intervention by addressing nutrition, physical activity, and preventive health care strategies. You can use these programs as examples to design, implement, and evaluate your own effective, engaging, and successful wellness initiatives or programs.

With escalating global health care costs and current economic challenges affecting all sectors of society, the time is right for worksites, communities, and schools to focus on wellness that works. Additionally, with a wider array of professions in unrelated disciplines and in varied settings taking interest in promoting health and wellness initiatives, *Winning Health Promotion Strategies* is a timely resource for those looking for up-to-date guidance, tools, best practices, and practical examples for winning health promotion initiatives.

Winning Health Promotion Strategies is also timely with the release of many U.S. federal, state, and local guidelines and initiatives, such as the release of the nation's first Physical Activity Guidelines for Americans by the U.S. Department of Health and Human Services in 2008 (www.health.gov/paguidelines/), the National Physical Activity Plan (www.physicalactivityplan.org/index.htm), and other recent health initiatives, such as First Lady Michelle Obama's *Let's Move* campaign: "America's Move to Raise a Healthier Generation of Kids" (www.letsmove.gov). *Winning Health Promotion Strategies* can provide programs, resources, strategies, and ideas to execute these important plans and initiatives in a wide variety of settings. The book is a toolbox of user-friendly tools and resources that facilitates the ongoing, successful, and collective growth of the wellness industry.

An Era of Change

Many of us are familiar with Albert Einstein's definition of insanity: doing the same thing over and over again and expecting different results. We know that change is needed in many sectors of our society, including the health and wellness industry. As health and wellness professionals, we need to change our approach to resolving mounting health care issues by changing the strategies we have traditionally employed to improve the lifestyle behaviors of millions of people. A saner approach is to take into account the many individual, societal, economic, and psychosocial influences on health behavior.

To do this, we need to rally together a village of multidisciplinary practitioners. We need to inspire individuals to become part of the solution to the escalating health care crisis by taking individual responsibility for health and lifestyle behaviors. If we truly want better health outcomes and health cost containment, we must change our approach by changing our thinking, and inspire others to lead healthy lives. *Winning Health Promotion Strategies* serves *multi*disciplinary practitioners who seek to overcome present-day challenges with an *inter*disciplinary approach that comprehensively draws from all areas of expertise.

"The global health economy is growing faster than gross domestic product (GDP), having increased its share from 8% to 8.6% of the world's GDP between 2000 and 2005. In absolute terms, adjusted for inflation, this represents a 35% growth in the world's expenditure on health over a five-year period" (World Health Report, 2008). Recently, more research has been conducted internationally in the wellness industry than ever before. Findings from this research have led to the creation and dissemination of a massive number of health education programs that have saturated the public through a wide range of channels. Nevertheless, the nutrition and physical activity practices of Americans have changed little, if at all, and the health care crisis and associated costs continue to escalate. Let's face it: We must change our current approach to health and wellness.

The most successful leaders I have met and worked with in the wellness industry consider the comprehensive influences on health. They have a satellite rather than microscopic view of the complex issues related to individual behavior change. They use the talent and expertise of multidisciplinary practitioners, as well as their clients, to design, implement, and evaluate their health and wellness initiatives. They seek to identify and understand determining factors of health and apply evidence-based strategies to behavior change. *Winning Health Promotion Strategies* provides broad insight into these important considerations and strategies for change to achieve successful outcomes, along with innovative and model health and wellness programs that may be implemented in worksite, community, and school settings.

An Era of Challenge

The health and wellness industry currently faces serious individual, societal, economic, and psychosocial issues. *Winning Health Promotion Strategies* takes these issues into account while providing tools for positive health behavior change. *Perceived* barriers to participation in health and wellness programs, in both practitioners and participants, become *real* barriers. Arguably, more perceived barriers to the practice of health and wellness exist now than in any other time in history. Addressing these barriers is just as important as using multidisciplinary, evidence-based guidelines and behavior change theories in the design, implementation, and evaluation of health and wellness programs.

One of the most common reported barriers to initiating and adhering to a healthy lifestyle is the decline of discretionary time. We live in a time-deprived society. Today, people are working longer hours. There are more dual-income families, more single-parent families, and more overcommitted schedules than ever before. Many people report that they would really like to practice a healthier lifestyle, but they just don't have the time. As a result, they put their health on the back burner to fulfill other pressing commitments and priorities. With conflicting priorities and a lack of discretionary time comes stress. With stress comes illness, and with illness comes elevated health care costs and a host of other psychosocial issues.

Elevated stress, chronic diseases, and related risk factors have translated into the continual escalation of global health care expenditures that impact *all* of us today. Results reported for a large, multi-employer, multi-site, employee population (the largest database of its kind assembled to date) identified seven of ten modifiable health risks significantly associated with higher health care expenditures over a short-term period (Goetzel, Anderson, Whitmer et al., 1998). This study demonstrated that individuals at high risk for poor health outcomes had significantly higher expenditures than did those at lower risk in seven of ten risk categories. Individuals who reported themselves as depressed incurred 70 percent higher health care expenditures, and those reported to be at high stress incurred 46 percent higher health care costs. Also, those employees who had high blood glucose, were extremely over or underweight, used tobacco, had high blood pressure, and led sedentary lifestyles incurred higher medical expenditures compared with those lacking these risks, even when all other risk factors were taken into account. In this study, "risk-free" individuals incurred average annual medical expenditures totaling $1,166; in comparison, "high-risk" individuals had average medical expenditures totaling $3,803, more than three times the cost of "risk-free" individuals. ("High-risk" individuals include those whose health habits and biometric measures put them at risk for heart disease because they smoked, did not exercise, ate poorly, were hypertensive, had high cholesterol, or reported being highly stressed.) Also noteworthy is that individuals who reported being both depressed and highly stressed were found to be 147 percent more costly than their counterparts without those risks, underscoring the impact of psychosocial factors on health and productivity. There also is a strong documented association between stress-related chronic fatigue and chronic disease and their related risk factors. Based on cross-sectional data analyzed from the second British National Survey of Psychiatric Morbidity (2000), chronic fatigue (significant reported fatigue lasting 6 months or more) is significantly associated with physical illness, even after adjusting or accounting for all sociodemographic and psychiatric factors (Watanabe, Steward, Jenkins et al., 2008).

There is a global epidemic of chronic disease emerging (https://apps.who.int/infobase/report.aspx). Chronic diseases, such as heart disease, stroke, cancer, chronic respiratory diseases, and diabetes, are the leading cause of mortality in the world, representing 60 percent of all deaths. In addition, out of the 35 million people worldwide who died from chronic disease in 2005, half were under age 70 and half were women (www.who.int/topics/chronic_diseases/en/). A global study of the burden of disease conducted by the World Health Organization, the World Bank, and Harvard

University revealed that mental illness, including suicide, accounts for more than 15 percent of the burden of disease in established market economies, such as the United States. This surpasses the disease burden caused by all cancers (Murray and Lopez, 1996).

The current weakened global economy translates into increased stress levels that affect our personal health behaviors. When faced with financial decisions, people lean toward less expensive options. Many times, healthy food choices and other healthy lifestyle practices, such as purchasing and using a fitness club or gym membership, are not perceived as economical. Simultaneously, however, 54 percent of workers are concerned about health problems caused by stress, and stress is associated with a lack of energy, inactivity, and sedentary behavior. As a result, many Americans find themselves living a vicious cycle. *Winning Health Promotion Strategies* addresses recommended practices from marketing and consumer behavior research to promote the reinvestment of discretionary time in healthy lifestyle practices.

Another challenge facing the health and wellness industry is related to the recent and continual exponential growth in technology. Our society has grown accustomed to instant gratification. We can communicate instantly. We can get food faster. We can get money faster. We can travel faster. Credit cards have provided us with the ability to purchase just about anything we want without having to wait until we have the cash. We don't like to wait. We tend to put off preventive maintenance of our homes and cars, and our health. We wait until things break or we become ill before addressing our problems, and then we seek quick solutions.

In this age of continually advancing technology, healthy lifestyle practices are not perceived as quick fixes to excess weight and acute or chronic diseases. The benefits and results of healthy lifestyle behaviors do not manifest themselves as quickly as microwave popcorn. The U.S. weight-loss industry has capitalized on this attitude and translated it into a $30-billion-a-year industry. Even in the midst of the current economic downturn, the global weight management market continues to grow and is estimated to reach US$586 billion in 2014 from about US$363 billion in 2009 (www.marketsandmarkets.com/Market-Reports/global-weight-loss-and-gain-market-research-28.html).

As health and wellness professionals, we are called to face the challenge of designing and delivering wellness programs for the individual consumer. Almost everyone has, at some point in their lives, gained or lost weight or battled an acute or chronic health condition. We must not address health and wellness using a one-size-fits-all approach. What works for me may not work for you, and vice versa. We are a very diverse global community not only in race and ethnicity, but also in age, gender, socioeconomic status, educational level, culture, geographic location, genetics, and personal preferences, among other factors. *Winning Health Promotion Strategies* will help design health and wellness programs for dissemination, and take all of these factors into account.

An Opportunity to Inspire!

Recently, following a panel presentation at the Wellness and Prevention Health Care Congress in Washington, DC, a close colleague introduced me to a man in the audience who was from my home state of Rhode Island. The man quickly responded to my colleague, "I know Annie, the Rock Star of Wellness!" We all laughed at this very interesting introduction. As the former director of the Governor's Wellness Initiative in Rhode Island, I had the opportunity to work with many representatives of the wellness industry in the smallest state in the union, as well as in states across the country. A rock star, however, I hardly thought!

Afterward, I realized there is much more to a rock star than notoriety. Rock stars *inspire* people. They have the ability to motivate and, in some cases, move people toward change through their craft. When many of us listen to a musician or rock star, we experience vivid memories of some of the most challenging, and joyous, times of our lives. Through their lyrics and inspiring performances, rock stars connect with millions of people and inspire some of them to make significant life-altering changes. Health and wellness professionals may learn a great deal from rock stars as they strive to inspire people to move toward positive change and engagement in healthy lifestyle behaviors.

Throughout my career in wellness (over the last three decades), I have had the privilege and pleasure of meeting and working with many rock stars of wellness. These colleagues have all applied their unique brand and style to their approach to health and wellness programs. They possess an uncanny ability to connect with people and motivate them to make significant health behavior changes and achieve positive health outcomes.

Like the entertainment business, the health and wellness industry is about engaging the audience. As we engage our audience in healthy lifestyle behaviors, we must also be diligent about the business side of the equation for optimal success. This means that we must take all the necessary behind-the-scenes steps to ensure that our health and wellness programs are steeped in scientific evidence and thoroughly planned, implemented, and evaluated with data to measure success and guide subsequent program design for a positive return on investment.

In the 1980s, I served as the Rhode Island representative of the International Dance Exercise Association (IDEA). At one of our international conference meetings, I attended a session called The Educated Entertainer. This session had a lasting impact on me and helped change my thinking on how to best deliver wellness to my clients. The notion of both *educating* and *entertaining* program participants so they sustain participation struck a chord within me. The health and wellness industry should not deliver wellness the way a traditional health care professional treats medical conditions. The health and wellness industry is charged with addressing identified health risks and delivering evidence-based programs in a fun and engaging manner, while keeping a pulse on the latest consumer-driven trends. Quite a balancing act! *Winning Health Promotion Strategies* provides you with the evidence-based tools needed to become your own rock star of wellness as you make a significant impact on keeping people healthy and reducing the burden of acute and chronic disease.

How to Use This Book

Part I of this book begins by revealing the wide range of opportunities that exist today for health and wellness professionals. The descriptions of a variety of settings will help individual wellness professionals, as well as wellness business owners, expand their services into different markets, increasing demand as well as revenues. For those who are implementing wellness initiatives in one particular setting, such as a community-based organization or worksite, or in multiple settings, chapter 1 provides a comprehensive perspective on the current health and wellness industry.

Chapter 2 provides a step-by-step outline of effective strategies for planning, launching, as well as sustaining, a winning health promotion initiative. This chapter provides stories, as well as a variety of examples, of organizations that have successfully implemented full-scale wellness initiatives over time.

Whether you are launching a few health improvement programs or a full-scale wellness initiative, motivation and engagement strategies are critical to maximize participation, positive health behavior change, and improved health outcomes in any population. Many unique and effective engagement strategies are presented in chapter 3. Strategies are based on evidence-based health behavior change theories and processes that may be applied to either populations or individuals.

Chapter 4 provides assessment and evaluation tools and steps to improve your existing wellness initiatives as well as strategies to take them to the next level. Sustaining a successful initiative is an evolutionary process, not a destination. This chapter presents ideas for building on existing wellness programs as well as strategies for improving, growing, and evaluating them.

Part I assists you with planning, launching, and sustaining the programs detailed in part II of this book. Application of the strategies presented in part I to any of the programs in part II will result in greater participation and improved health outcomes.

Part II features 55 winning health promotion programs. Depending on your goals, you may use part II to create a single program, several programs, or a full-scale wellness initiative. These model programs may also support other less visible wellness programs such as online health improvement or telephonic coaching programs designed to strengthen the culture of wellness in any setting.

Although many of the 55 programs presented in part II may be implemented in worksite, community, or school settings, each includes icons indicating the most appropriate setting(s) for implementation. Also, each program is categorized by program type: awareness, education, or intervention. An activity finder is also included after the table of contents to help you easily locate programs by health topic such as physical activity, nutrition, and general health or preventive tools.

The 55 programs follow a set structure, making it easy for you to find pertinent information. Every program contains some, if not all, of the following features:

Icons identify the different characteristics of each program.

The introduction provides a quick summary of the program.

Goals are presented for each program.

The description details the premise of the program and provides other information on how the program should be run.

Some programs outline special equipment and supplies that are needed in order to successfully run the program.

Enhancements provide ideas for how you can modify a program to suit your needs.

Contact information is provided so you can receive additional information, program supplies, or support.

Some programs contain examples of handouts you can provide for your participants.

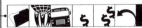

An Apple a Day

An Apple a Day is a nutrition intervention program. Participants who eat an apple each day at work, school, or a community-based organization such as a community center or health club for 21 consecutive days receive an incentive such as a raffle ticket.

Goals

- Increase apple (fruit) consumption.
- Educate participants on the benefits of eating apples (fruit).

Description   A bushel of shiny, delicious apples is prominently displayed on a table next to the front desk, and employees are encouraged to take one each day for the month of September. (Contact local orchards to obtain discounted rates on apples, or encourage participants to bring their own apple in each day.) Employees get Apple a Day cards punched each day they eat an apple. (See the bottom of this page for a punch card you can use.) At the end of the 21 days, anyone who hands in a completed punch card is entered into a raffle. Apple recipes are also provided each week to help employees continue eating apples by providing a variety of options for preparing or cooking with apples. This type of intervention is effective because it reinforces education (i.e., learning about the benefits of apple consumption) with the desired behavior change (i.e., increased apple consumption).

Enhancements

- Contact local registered dietitians or nutritionists in private practice or at your state or local health departments or universities, or contact your local culinary college or any college in your area that offers a culinary arts program, for handouts on the benefits of eating apples and other fruits and vegetables, recipes, or on-site cooking demonstrations.
- Recipe boards may be hung in various locations for participants to share apple recipes.
- This program may be just a one-day awareness event at which apples, recipes, and handouts on their health benefits are distributed.

For More Information   Visit www.fruitsandveggiesmatter.gov/ to read about the benefits of eating apples (fruit) and for creative recipes.

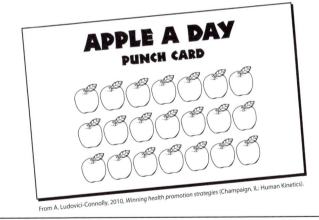

From A. Ludovici-Connolly, 2010, *Winning health promotion strategies* (Champaign, IL: Human Kinetics).

If you are interested in submitting a case study or wellness program for a potential sequel, please submit to annie@uri.edu.

First, my heartfelt thanks and love go out to my family.

To my son, Kyle, who is the light of my life and makes me proud to be his mother every day. Kyle, you have gown up to become a kind, talented, witty, and handsome young man. I know your father is proudly watching over you. To my husband, Greg Belanger, my best friend and trusted advisor. Greg, you are truly a renaissance man, continually providing me with invaluable insights and wisdom. Thank you both for your patience and ongoing support during this long journey of writing, researching, and publishing this book. I promise I WILL cook again!

To my mom, who started me on my motivational reading journey by reading books to me and my late brother, Dino, such as *The Little Train That Could* and *Hope for the Flowers.* Mom, you always encouraged us to follow our dreams and always provided us with the confidence to go after them.

Special thanks to my late grandparents, Avó and Avóa, who were like my second parents and also provided my start in the industry by being my "angel investors" in my first business venture, the Wakefield Health and Fitness Center.

To my Uncle Ed Pereira, artist and graphic designer extraordinaire, who helped me to develop countless book proposals, along with stunning book covers to market them. Finally, all our work paid off! I can't thank you enough for your help and support over the years.

And, to my late first husband and father of our son, Kyle; Mark J. Connolly. Mark also left this world, and all of us, way too soon, but showed incredible strength and courage throughout his battle with cancer. Mark taught many the meaning of true strength, that health *is* the greatest wealth, that life is short, and how to strive to make each and every day count.

Thank you to all my cousins, other family members, friends, and neighbors for being patient and understanding while I was in "hibernation" on nights and weekends writing. I look forward to seeing and socializing with all of you again real soon!

A very special thank you to my friend, colleague, and personal editor, Dr. Kathleen Cullinen. Kathy, your expertise, advice, guidance, and editorial direction have been invaluable. I can't thank you enough for your commitment and contributions to this project. Your edits, additions, and suggestions have completed this book, like icing on a cake!

A big thanks to my acquisitions editor, Myles Schrag, who saw something in my originally rejected book proposal. Myles, you had the vision and believed in this project before it was even launched. I will always be grateful for this opportunity to share my passion for wellness with such a large audience. Thank you to Amanda Ewing, my developmental editor, for polishing the structure and making the book shine even brighter! Thanks to everyone at Human Kinetics who had a hand in the publication of this book. You are exemplary of the collaborative and dedicated teamwork described in this book!

I would also like to offer special acknowledgments to the governor of Rhode Island, the Honorable Donald L. Carcieri, and his lovely wife, First Lady Suzanne Carcieri. I am grateful to you for putting your trust in me and providing me with the invaluable opportunity to lead Get Fit, Rhode Island! I will always appreciate your personal and executive support of Get Fit. I will never forget what we all accomplished for our great state and how much fun we had in the process!

To the wellness champions of Rhode Island: Wow, what a ride! I cannot tell you all how much I enjoyed working with all of you. Thank you to the first champions for "hitting the beach" with me as we launched the initiative together. We certainly earned our battle wounds the first couple of years! To all who joined along the way, thank you for reenergizing us as you joined our wellness family.

Thank you to everyone in the governor's office, including those in the scheduling, health policy, legislative, and press secretary offices, for all the support you provided to Get Fit over the years. Special thanks to Cheryl Martone for your hard work and support.

Sincere thanks to everyone at the University of Rhode Island who supported me and Get Fit, especially vice president and former congressman, Robert Weygand. Bob, I will always appreciate everything you have done for me. Thanks to Laura Kenerson, director of personnel, and all of my friends in human resources.

I also want to thank my academic mentors at the University of Rhode Island, including Dr. Bob Comerford of the College of Business, who fueled my interest in business and who provided his guidance and counsel as I purchased and launched my health club. Thanks to Dr. Albert Della Bitta, from the University of Rhode Island's College of Business, for instilling in me the power and value of marketing in all industries, including health and wellness. Thanks to Dr. Tom Manfredi for encouraging me to pursue my master's degree in kinesiology and for providing me with my first teaching and research opportunities at the university.

I especially want to thank Dr. James Prochaska for the honor to serve as a scholar in residence at the Cancer Research Prevention Center at the University of Rhode Island. I will always appreciate your insights and valuable edits and contributions to this book, as well as the opportunity to continue to collaborate with you and everyone on your research team.

I also want to thank Jim Winkler, health management practice leader for Hewitt, for taking the time to write the foreword for this book and for providing superior executive support for wellness at Hewitt Associates.

To all of my colleagues and friends old and new, unfortunately too numerous to thank here, with whom I have had the pleasure of working with over the past three decades—I have truly enjoyed my journey in this industry with each and every one of you!

Last but not least, to all who shared their programs, research, personal experiences, and successes with me. You all have helped make this book what it is, and I appreciate your contributions, your friendship, and your support!

Yours in Health,
Anne Marie Ludovici-Connolly-Belanger

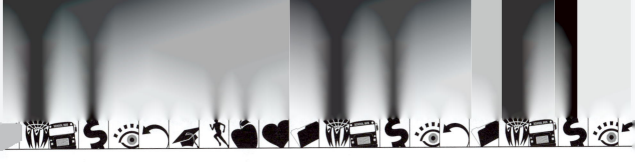

Understanding Wellness Initiatives

Part I of this book provides a framework for developing a comprehensive wellness initiative, as well as innovative strategies to increase engagement in single, stand-alone wellness programs. This part begins by discussing the variety of settings in which health and wellness initiatives are being implemented. Chapter 1 (Making Wellness Work in Various Settings) offers health and wellness practitioners suggestions on where and how to market your services and programs to enhance revenue and grow client base by presenting the rationale for implementing wellness strategies in a variety of settings. If you are working in one particular setting, such as a worksite, this information may be useful as you seek additional resources within and outside of your industry or setting to support your efforts. Chapter 2 (Developing Successful Wellness Initiatives) lays out effective, comprehensive, and evidence-based strategies for designing, implementing, and evaluating your wellness initiative or program using a step-by-step approach. Chapter 3 (Creating Engaging Wellness Initiatives) details creative strategies for engaging your target population and provides practical examples for applying evidence-based behavior change theories and techniques to engage and sustain the active engagement of your target audience over time. Finally, chapter 4 (Improving and Expanding Existing Wellness Initiatives) may appeal to readers with more mature or seasoned wellness initiatives by discussing strategies for maintaining and sustaining the growth of wellness initiatives or programs, return on investment (ROI), and positive health outcomes. All chapters provide real-world examples from model and proven wellness initiatives and programs, evidence-based practices, and advice from experts in the wellness industry.

You may read the chapters in part I in the order presented or refer to them on an ongoing, individual basis depending on your needs, interests, and goals. In summary, part I provides a detailed explanation of the components and step-by-step approaches necessary to develop new wellness initiatives or to enhance existing wellness initiatives in worksite, community, or school settings. Part I also includes engagement strategies that you can apply to your existing wellness programs or any of the model programs presented in part II of this book.

Making
Wellness Work
in Various Settings

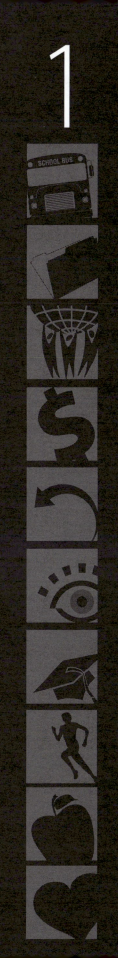

Intraoffice Memo

Topic: Mandatory meeting

Where: First-floor conference room

When: September 15

Time: 11:00 a.m. to 12:00 p.m.

Note: This will be a walking meeting. Please wear comfortable shoes and bring a water bottle.

At Salo, LLC, a financial staffing corporation of 50 employees based in Minnesota, treadmill workstations (see Moving Meetings in part II) have replaced the large conference table. Meetings are now, literally, working meetings—actually, working-out meetings! Yes, the employees actually walk at a slow pace on their treadmills as they meet.

If you read the preceding memo a few years ago, you may have thought the note section was an error or even a joke. Not today. Health and wellness professionals are witnessing "out of the box" thinking about the delivery of health promotion in a variety of ways and settings. This example demonstrates that there is a wave of employers now incorporating unusual, and very unconventional, healthy practices into many aspects of the workday, including meetings. Worksites have not only incorporated wellness into their workdays, but they have also incorporated wellness into their *work*! Employers with limited budgets or who are not ready to invest in equipment, such as treadmill workstations, are instituting policies allowing employees to conduct walking meetings. Small groups of employees can opt to walk outdoors to meet as opposed to sitting in offices. These types of innovative approaches to wellness are also occurring in communities and schools.

As health care costs continue to climb, individuals, families, communities, employers, and governments face serious financial challenges to sustain basic health care coverage. The costs associated with overweight, obesity, and related chronic diseases are at an all-time high and climbing. Chronic diseases and related conditions are now the major cause of death and disability worldwide. The annual impact on the U.S. economy of the most common chronic diseases is calculated to be more than $1 trillion, which could increase to nearly $6 trillion by the middle of this century.

Across the world, expenditure on health is also growing. Between 1995 and 2005, spending almost doubled—from $2.6 to $5.1 trillion. Additionally, this rate of growth is accelerating. Between 2000 and 2005, the total amount spent on health throughout the world increased by $330 billion on average each year, against an average of $197 billion in each of the five previous years. In fact, health expenditure is growing faster than both GDP and population growth (World Health Organization, 2010).

Health professionals can leverage this crisis by offering wellness programs that can improve the health and quality of life of individuals and decrease health care costs. The latter is a very appealing motivator for senior-level leadership to support a wellness initiative.

Wellness is now recognized as a respected part of the solution to the global health care crisis. The 2008 U.S. presidential candidates listed prevention, programs or initiatives, and wellness among their top strategies for controlling escalating health care costs. There is a growing demand, in a variety of venues, for wellness programs that work. The increasing need for effective programs has created a greater demand for sound resources. This book is written not only for health and wellness professionals who are interested in starting wellness programs, but also for those interested in taking existing, successful or perhaps mediocre, wellness programs to the next level.

Health and wellness promotion strategies have proven to be effective in the most obvious and unobvious places, in the most obvious and unobvious ways, providing new opportunities for health professionals. Many of these opportunities were never available before. The time is ripe for health promotion and wellness—catch the wave! By reengineering their thinking and expanding their products, services, and markets for employers, government officials, municipalities, and schools, health and wellness professionals are gaining additional exposure in their communities and profits to their bottom lines. In addition, health and wellness professionals are offering on-site services as well as discounts for in-house programs and services for large groups. In many cases, worksites, communities, and schools are contracting with outside vendors and industry professionals to support or enhance their wellness initiatives and programs.

This chapter covers the various settings in which wellness may be promoted, including worksites, communities, and schools. It is important to realize the wide range of opportunity for wellness promotion in order to understand the scope of its potential impact on public, as well as individual, health. Part II describes programs that may be offered in each of these settings and for each of these populations. Some programs are targeted for specific settings such as schools, but many may be offered in multiple settings.

Tip

If you are a health and wellness professional looking to build your client base or revenue, here are some steps that you can take to build, expand, or enhance wellness programs or services:

- List employers in your area that could benefit from your services.
- Contact local health insurers to see whether they hire wellness experts.
- Check to see whether your state, provincial, or local government offers a wellness program for its employees. Offer to get involved.
- Find out whether your school district has a wellness committee that you may join. If not, write to the superintendent and offer to start one.
- Review health and wellness programs offered by your local parks and recreation department.
- Locate or compile a directory of community wellness programs.

The National Governors Association Healthy America Initiative

The National Governors Association (NGA) Healthy America initiative is a call to action for states to support wellness for all citizens. Governor Mike Huckabee of Arkansas declared wellness a priority during his term as chair of the NGA and launched the Healthy America initiative in 2005. Healthy America encouraged state governors to launch "wellness where we work, live, and learn" and to work alongside the NGA to improve the health of children and adults in an effort to address the health care crisis. Healthy America challenged governors to promote wellness in a wide range of venues, from worksites, schools, municipalities, and hospitals, to communities and faith-based organizations. Since the beginning of this initiative, many states have launched health and wellness promotion initiatives and programs, reaching diverse populations and large numbers of people (www.nga.org). (While this is a U.S.-based initiative, the idea behind it and the outcome of it are applicable around the world.)

At the 2007 NGA Healthy States Summit, over 30 state representatives shared success stories related to their progress on the Healthy States program, a component of the Healthy America initiative. In response to the 2005 call to action, a variety of states and locations offering wellness programs reported on the details of their programs that were yielding results. I was fortunate to have represented Rhode Island at this meeting and to have witnessed the creative, outstanding health promotion programs being implemented across the United States. Clearly, much progress has been made under the leadership of the health policy team at the NGA and governors across the country. Many states are hiring outside consultants and vendors and engaging in public–private partnerships to accomplish their wellness goals. Examples of effective wellness programs being launched across the country are highlighted throughout this book.

The NGA identified three priority areas for states to include:

Wellness where we work

Wellness where we live

Wellness where we learn

The NGA's three priority areas align nicely with the nation's first National Physical Activity Plan (NPAP) (www.physicalactivityplan.org/index.htm).

According to the Web site, "The National Plan aims to create a culture that supports physically active lifestyles for the ultimate purposes of improving health, preventing disease and disability, and enhancing quality of life." Additionally, the National Physical Activity Plan aligns with other relevant initiatives across the United States. In an effort to empower all Americans to be physically active, the plan is a proud strategic partner with a comprehensive network of organizations and resources, including First Lady Michelle Obama's *Let's Move* campaign.

Eight sectors have been identified to work collaboratively to execute the plan (www.physicalactivityplan.org/sectors/index.htm). These eight sectors include:

1. Public health
2. Education
3. Volunteer and non-profit organizations
4. Transportation, urban design, and community planning
5. Mass media
6. Healthcare
7. Business and industry
8. Parks, recreation, fitness, and sports

Resources, including white papers, for the channels addressed in this book (worksites, communities, and schools) are available through the National Physical Activity Plan. Part II of this book provides programs that can assist with execution of the National Plan in your setting.

The rest of this chapter outlines how you can use these three settings, or channels, to implement wellness programs.

Get Fit, Rhode Island! A Governor's Call to Action

In 2005, Rhode Island governor, Donald L. Carcieri, formally launched Get Fit, Rhode Island!, a state employee wellness initiative, and declared a statewide goal for Rhode Island to become the first well state in the nation, a designation awarded by the Wellness Council of America (WELCOA). To achieve WELCOA's well state status, more than 20 percent of all Rhode Island's employees had to be offered wellness programs at work. This aggressive goal required a collaborative spirit, public–private partnerships, and the active senior leadership and support of Governor Carcieri and the First Lady of Rhode Island, Suzanne Carcieri, to achieve success. Rhode Island businesses, government leaders, and health officials rallied and put aside political and competitive interests for the achievement of a common goal. In 2007, Rhode Island became the first well state in the nation.

The University of Rhode Island, under the leadership of Robert Weygand, the vice president of administration and finance and a former U.S. congressman, and Dr. David Gifford, the director of the state health department, oversaw Get Fit, Rhode Island! (Get Fit). Beside a front line of bright, passionate, and personable employees from each of 25 state departments appointed to serve as the state's wellness champions, I proudly served as the director of Get Fit for three years. The commitment of the wellness champions, detailed in chapter 2, was critical to the success of Get Fit. The program also used the expertise of state departments and community-based organizations to mobilize the wellness initiative.

The Worksite Wellness Council of Rhode Island (WWCRI) championed Rhode Island's well state recognition by WELCOA by recruiting and assisting more than 250 public and private businesses throughout the state with their certification processes. To accomplish the state's wellness mission, collaborative relationships were forged among state and industry leaders, including the top health insurers in the state. Michael Samuelson, senior vice president of Blue Cross Blue Shield of Rhode Island, joined the WWCRI arrival to Rhode Island in 2003 and provided his expertise and resources to assist in achieving the well state goal. UnitedHealthcare of New England's CEO, Stephen Farrell, also stepped up and fully supported Rhode Island's well state efforts.

Through collaborations and senior-level support, Rhode Island achieved success.

Priority 1: Wellness Where We Work

Health care has soared to the top of almost every CEO's agenda as health care costs continue to rise globally. Along with health care costs, the workweek continues to increase steadily, with the average now being more than 50 hours. These trends have resulted in support for worksite wellness. Organizations can glean numerous benefits from wellness programs. The return on investment (ROI) of wellness progress is threefold: for every dollar invested in wellness, three dollars are saved. Worksite wellness translates into the following:

Tip

If you represent a worksite, community, or school seeking to launch or enhance a wellness initiative, see chapters 2 and 3, respectively, for more information on strategies for success.

- Reduction of documented perceived barriers (e.g., time, energy, resources)
- Stress reduction
- Improved social support of colleagues, improving exercise adherence
- Improved job satisfaction and morale (e.g., positive water cooler talk)
- Improved employer–employee relations (e.g., mayor walking with employees)
- Positive public opinion of elected officials

With the increase in dual-income families and the increase in the average workweek, many people have less discretionary time than ever before. Delivering wellness at work just makes sense and translates into lower health care costs, benefit savings, and improved quality of life for employees. Employers, large and small, have observed the numerous benefits that worksite wellness programs offer. Providing social support and time savings, wellness programs at the worksite appear to be a natural fit for successfully engaging adults in healthy lifestyle practices.

This perceived barrier of discretionary time has increased the demand for the convenience of worksite-based health promotion and wellness programs. As people spend more time at work, it makes sense to engage them where they are, making healthy lifestyles convenient and affordable at a place where they can receive social support and recognition or incentives for positive lifestyle changes. The following strategies and tips may assist you in developing effective worksite wellness programs:

• **Self-directed programs.** Self-directed programs have been proven to be effective because employees can have difficulty attending a class or event at a specific time. Such programs allow employees to be engaged at their own pace, on their own time, and at various levels of involvement.

• **Short-duration programs.** Educational workshops that are 15 to 30 minutes long attract more employees than longer ones do. If necessary, you can deliver more content over a series of workshops.

• **Workday programs.** Providing programs during work hours increases participation. If allowed to participate on company time, such as during breaks or lunch, even more employees attend.

• **Programs with incentives.** Incentives have been shown to increase participation in worksite wellness programs and initiatives, particularly when linked to health benefit credits such as a reduction of health insurance copayments. However, the affect of incentives on financial outcomes remains unclear. Incentives are discussed in chapter 3.

- **Programs with top-down and bottom-up support.** The support of senior leadership, middle management, and frontline employees, or ground troops, is a must. Even when senior leadership is on board, middle management may take additional recruitment efforts due to demanding workloads. Middle management, to whom the majority of employees directly report, needs to be supportive of employee participation in wellness events or meetings during normal business hours when possible. It is important that senior management and middle management openly discuss and address any supports and barriers to implementing a wellness initiative. It is also imperative that support come from the bottom up through peer and social networks (see chapter 3).

To reach the largest number of employees in a worksite setting, consider offering wellness programs at all locations, including remote or satellite locations, and during multiple work shifts. Worksite wellness programming must be sensitive to the time demands of employees as well as employers. Shorter programs may be an effective way to provide a taste of what a longer, more comprehensive initiative may entail. Programs offered at lunchtime are often better attended than those offered after work because many employees do not want to stay at their worksites after the workday has ended. Break time can be a good time to offer snapshots of health promotion opportunities. Wellness information and programs may be delivered to offices on mail carts to maximize participation, especially of the busiest executives.

Priority 2: Wellness Where We Live

On warm summer evenings on the streets of Nashville, Tennessee, you can get a great workout, along with dance lessons, engage in live music, and meet enthusiastic people at weekly summer dance block parties. Nashville's Metro Parks and Recreation Department hosts these dance parties for eight consecutive weeks. Each week a different band is featured, providing music for all ages. Dance lessons are provided for community members. This gives the community an opportunity to gather, socialize, and exercise.

In a Nashville senior center, *Let's Dance*, a one-hour dance class (featured in part II), attracted more participants than any physical activity program previously offered. The senior center had advertised many exercise classes in the past, only to draw minimal participation, until Let's Dance. This class had great appeal!

These examples demonstrate that girls and boys and men and women of all ages "just wanna have fun." Dancing not only is a great physical activity program, but it also has a therapeutic social component, which fosters self-efficacy, or self-confidence in adopting healthy lifestyle behaviors. (Bandura's self-efficacy theory is discussed in chapter 3.) Communities, municipalities, and faith-based organizations are recognizing the need for members to practice healthy lifestyle behaviors. Of all the environments we move through, there may be no better place to achieve a healthy lifestyle than our own communities.

Communities have a unique opportunity to influence large populations; they have a captive audience and therefore can uniquely engage families, where they reside, in healthy lifestyle behaviors and programs. Communities may also have a variety of resources at their disposal to assist in wellness efforts, including departments such as buildings and grounds, recreation, and other municipal departments. These departments and their employees may have resources, services, budgets, and contacts, as well as unique perspectives and ideas, that can be leveraged to execute wellness programs.

How do wellness strategies in communities differ from other settings? How can you maximize results? Here are a few tips for success:

- Plan events that can easily accommodate large groups of people.
- Offer wellness opportunities for families.
- Take advantage of seasonal sports and activities. For example, offer snowshoeing or ice skating in the winter, and offer walking programs and dance lessons in the summer.
- Partner with other groups such as nonprofit organizations, other municipalities, and state departments.
- Advocate for effective policy and environmental changes to support healthy behaviors (see chapter 4).
- Arrange social opportunities to encourage commitment of participants in wellness activities.

Tip

To implement a winning wellness program or initiative in a variety of settings, you may need to call on experts from a variety of disciplines. For example, a registered dietitian may be needed for on-site nutrition classes. For biometric screenings, a registered nurse will be required. Once you have determined the focus of your programming efforts and strategy, discussed in chapter 2, you will have a better idea of the expertise necessary to carry out your strategy. A comprehensive on-site initiative may require specialists from the following areas:

- Alternative therapies
- Corporate management
- Exercise physiology
- Health education
- Human resources
- Martial arts
- Massage therapy
- Nursing
- Nutrition
- Personal training
- Psychology
- Recreation, sports, and dance

Priority 3: Wellness Where We Learn

"Yuck! Look at all the germs, and I just washed my hands!," the middle school girl declared to her friends. As students observed their hands in a dark box after applying Glo Germ, they were able to see the millions of germs remaining after hand washing prior to entering the lunchroom. At an annual Kick Colds and Flu campaign (featured in part II) to reduce the spread of flu and the common cold, faculty and staff may pick up information and giveaways and participate in hands-on demonstrations to increase children's knowledge and change their hand-washing habits to minimize the spread of germs.

Schools and universities recognize the opportunity and obligation to promote healthy minds and bodies through offering wellness programs to faculty, staff, and students where they spend most of their waking hours—at school. Featuring changes in policies, wellness programs, and conventional health and gym classes, schools are building a menu of wellness initiatives. Many schools are now developing wellness committees that include representatives from local government, nonprofit organizations, private businesses, parents, and teachers, among others.

First Lady Michelle Obama has assembled a new interagency task force that will develop a comprehensive plan of action to combat the growing obesity epidemic in children. Like the NGA Healthy America initiative, the National Physical Activity Plan (NPAP), and Get Fit, Rhode Island!, Obama's *Let's Move* campaign will take a comprehensive, interdisciplinary approach, and engage both the private and public sectors. The goal of the campaign is to, "help children become more active and eat healthier within a generation, so that children born today will reach adulthood at a healthy weight" (www.whitehouse.gov/blog/2010/02/09/making-moves-a-healthier-generation).

Let's Move provides solutions and challenges for healthy schools, such as the Healthier US Schools Challenge Program (www.letsmove.gov/schools/index.html). In addition to the abundance of resources provided to promote healthy schools, *Let's Move* also provides solutions to enhance access to improve nutrition and physical activity, along with many resources to promote healthy homes and communities (www.letsmove.gov/).

Call your local school district to see whether it has a wellness committee. If it does, join. If your district does not have a wellness committee, start one! How? Write to your superintendent and offer to organize such a committee. Identify key people involved in wellness in the community, and invite them to a meeting to discuss organizing a committee to improve the health and wellness of faculty, staff, and students.

Although academic success is strongly linked with health, increased academic pressures on school officials have prompted the request for more classroom time for academics, resulting in less time for physical education, physical activity, and recess. Competing demands for time pose barriers to wellness where we learn. Health-risk behaviors such as poor nutrition, physical inactivity, substance use, and violence are consistently linked to academic failure because they often affect students' school attendance, ability to pay attention in class, grades, and test scores. In turn, school funding is based, in part, on the overall academic performance of the school. Today, we are challenged with the need to embed health into the education environment for all students. One solution to improving health and academic performance is short-duration programs. These may be creative, educational, and trendy, and they can engage parents via take-home materials.

Integration into the academic curriculum may be another solution for promoting wellness where we learn. As adults spend a majority of their waking hours at the worksite, children spend the majority of their waking hours at school. Lesson plans in other subjects can include wellness education. For example, history class can include physical activity by going on historical walks, or math lessons can integrate nutrition concepts. Teachers can get creative with coupling wellness education with a variety of topics. ABC for Fitness and Nutrition Detectives, featured in part II, are just two model programs that effectively integrate wellness into the school curriculum.

How do wellness strategies at schools differ from other settings? How can you maximize results? Here are a few tips for success:

- Integrate wellness education throughout the curriculum.
- Institute effective wellness policies that are easy to implement.
- Offer wellness information and displays during lunchtime.
- Offer interactive demonstrations to capture interest and attention.
- Offer take-home brochures to engage and involve parents.
- Offer programs to both students and staff.

Opportunities to Implement Successful Wellness Strategies

Following is an expanded list of settings in which to implement the NGA's three wellness priorities. As you have read, the opportunities are vast, the time is right, and resources are available to build successful wellness programs. Check this list as you spread the wealth of wellness!

Wellness Where We Work

Human resources organizations
Municipalities
Organized labor
Private sector worksites
Local, state, and federal government worksites

Wellness Were We Live

City or town recreation departments
Community health centers
Faith-based organizations
Health clubs and fitness centers
Hospitals
Nonprofit organizations
Nursing homes
Senior centers
Senior housing

Wellness Where We Learn

Early childhood centers
Schools
Universities and colleges

Summary

Health promotion programs and strategies work for a variety of people in a wide range of settings and occupations. This chapter details the types of settings in which wellness programs have been successful and describes the variety of professionals who are implementing wellness programs among various populations. The NGA identified three areas on which states should focus their attention: where we work, where we live, and where we learn. Other federal and state entities, such as the NPAP and *Let's Move* campaign, support this focus. Teachers, community recreation directors, public health and other health care professionals, business owners, and human resources staff, among others, may benefit from the strategies detailed throughout this book.

Developing Successful Wellness Initiatives

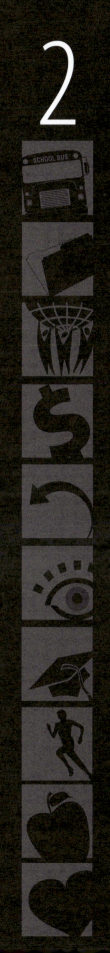

When the city of Gainesville, Florida, decided to pursue the title of the first well city in the United States, a prestigious designation awarded by the Wellness Council of America, Debbie Lee, cochair of the initiative's steering committee and marketing director for the Gainesville Health and Fitness Club, realized they needed more than great programs in order to achieve their wellness goals. The city needed to rally together, recruit an army of wellness "champions" to spread the word and excitement, craft a targeted strategy with goals, and orchestrate a wellness movement. Gainesville created a tight strategic plan and effective wellness programs using all of the evidence-based criteria required for success. However, city leaders also knew they needed to mobilize a large community of people; they needed to engage and inspire an entire city—and they did!

Gainesville had great leadership support for the effort. The mayor and the president of the chamber of commerce were on board, along with many local hospitals and business leaders. Additionally, Gainesville had the leadership of Debbie Lee, whose infectious enthusiasm inspired this army of volunteers to make the initiative a reality. Gainesville became the first well city in the United States.

Developing a wellness initiative should be approached in the same way as developing a new business or launching a special project within your workplace, community, or school. A well-thought-out written strategic operating plan, the allocation of adequate resources, and a high degree of attention and focus, along with inspiration from the top down and the bottom up, are required in order to realize positive outcomes. Success does not come swiftly or easily. It takes work, and it takes time. The sustained effort, commitment, and enthusiasm of an army of believers will move a wellness initiative forward. This chapter outlines some of the steps needed for implementing a wellness program or initiative.

Where to Begin

An organization was experiencing the worst financial climate in a decade. Employee morale was low, many jobs were being eliminated, and all department budgets were being cut. Leaders began investigating possible savings options within all divisions of the organization, including health care costs. To help accomplish this goal, they were contemplating the implementation of an employee wellness initiative. They were interested but not sure if they were fully committed to the idea. The director of human resources asked, "If we were to offer a wellness initiative, where would we begin?" Where would you begin? First, consider the following questions:

1. **What are your goals for wellness?** If your goal is to introduce wellness to the organization, then you may want to begin by offering one or two wellness programs (see program examples in part II). If the goal is to make a significant impact on the culture and health of the organization, reduce health care costs and other costs such as

10 Themes of Health and Productivity Management (HPM)

In a study published by the Journal of Occupational and Environmental Medicine, Ron Goetzel and colleagues (2001) studied 43 employers and almost 1 million workers. The study established key performance measures, benchmarks, and best practices. The authors identified the following 10 themes of initiatives that have had financial success:

1. HPM is aligned with the overall business strategy of the organization.
2. There is an interdisciplinary team focus.
3. There is a champion or a team of champions.
4. Senior management and business operations are key members of the team.
5. Prevention, health promotion, and wellness staff are heavily embedded in HPM processes.
6. Emphasis is on quality-of-life improvement, not just cost cutting.
7. Data collection, measurement, reporting, evaluation, and return on investment studies are key to determining the effectiveness and performance of programs over time.
8. There is constant organization-wide communication.
9. There is a consistent need to improve by learning from others.
10. The team always has fun in the process.

How to incorporate these themes into a comprehensive wellness initiative will be discussed throughout part I of this book.

workers' compensation or sick days, or achieve any other significant outcomes, begin planning for a comprehensive wellness initiative.

2. **What are your resources?** If your resources and budget are slim, you may still offer a comprehensive wellness initiative, but you must be creative about using all of your current internal as well as external resources. Another option is to launch programs in phases over a period of time, or offer a few programs detailed in part II and wait until you can devote the funds and staff to make a bigger splash.

3. **How committed is the organization?** If the organization and its leadership are fully committed to wellness, a comprehensive initiative may be successful. If the commitment is low, beginning with a few programs until you can garner full support may be the way to go.

4. **What is the climate of the organization at this time?** Timing is everything. If it is a turbulent time within the organization, you may have a difficult time launching a comprehensive initiative. It really depends on many factors such as how the program is positioned and the commitment and goals of the organization.

There is no right or wrong direction in which to go based on how you answer these questions. You must use your best judgment and do what's best for your organization or group. The right answer for one organization may not be the right one for another. The wellness team or board of advisors should weigh all the internal and external variables when contemplating the timing of a program launch. Here are two strategies to choose from:

1. **Comprehensive wellness initiative:** This chapter can assist those who would like to create a comprehensive wellness initiative. The evidence-based steps to building a successful initiative are easy to follow and highly effective.

2. **Traditional wellness programming:** Another option for exploring wellness is to begin with a program or two. If you not quite ready or able to commit the time and resources to a full-scale initiative, begin with traditional programming to test the waters. Traditional programming may create some interest in wellness, reveal how open participants might be to a more comprehensive program, and provide time to get the support needed for a comprehensive initiative. Such programming also does not require intensive commitments such as employee health surveys. It is important to note that a return on investment (ROI) or organizational cost savings as a result of positive health behavior changes are less frequently observed with traditional programming.

Tips

- If you want to begin by offering only one or two wellness programs, you may choose from the menu of programs in part II of this book.
- If you already have a successful wellness initiative in place, but would like to enhance, modify, or adapt it to achieve even more success or reach a larger audience, see chapter 4.
- If you are going to launch a comprehensive wellness initiative or are looking to improve your existing program, keep reading.

Five Steps to Building a Successful Wellness Initiative

The five steps described in this section reflect the Wellness Council of America (WELCOA) benchmarks of best practices in health and wellness promotion (www.welcoa.org/) as well as research on health promotion from other reputable sources such as *ACSM's Worksite Health Promotion Manual* (Cox, 2003) and *Worksite Health Promotion* (Chenoweth, 2007). These evidence-based steps may be applied in worksite, community, and school settings.

When developing a comprehensive wellness initiative, think of the following five steps that spell out the word **IDEAS**:

Infrastructure: Building the internal foundation to sustain a wellness initiative

Data: Collecting data or information

Evaluation: Evaluating data, setting goals, and developing a strategic work plan

AEI programming: Developing, implementing, and evaluating awareness, education, and intervention programs

Success: Measuring, monitoring, and reporting your successes and lessons learned

Once you decide to launch a comprehensive wellness initiative, you should follow each of the steps in a timely manner. The important thing is not to lose momentum by waiting too long between steps, particularly between data collection and programming. Following a health risk survey or questionnaire (HRQ) to guide your overall strategic plan and programming, you should quickly begin the strategic planning phase and program implementation to maintain participant interest.

Step 1: Infrastructure—Building the Foundation to Sustain a Wellness Initiative

To sustain a wellness initiative, several key positions must be in place within the organization, and the people in those positions must be committed to building a strong infrastructure. Experts agree that senior leaders (the school principal, mayor, CEO, or governor) are the foundational support needed for launching and developing a successful wellness initiative.

Another person of primary importance is the wellness director, manager, or coordinator. This person focuses solely on providing the attention that a successful wellness initiative requires. The wellness director is the glue that keeps the initiative together, setting the strategic direction of the initiative, implementing its programs, and performing operational duties. The director keeps senior leadership informed of progress as well as what is needed for the initiative to thrive.

In addition, dedicated wellness champions are needed in order to infiltrate the organization. The wellness champions assist the director by attending meetings related to the direction and planning of the initiative and its programs, overcoming barriers, and promoting the initiative throughout the organization.

An advisory board or steering committee is also very helpful for providing senior-level direction and support for the initiative. The advisory board or steering committee consists of senior leadership and the wellness director, and may include one or two wellness champions and other high-level people in the organization who can assist with planning, providing resources, removing barriers, and tracking financial return on investment.

The following sections detail some of these critical positions.

Senior Leadership Support

In 2005, the governor of Rhode Island, the Honorable Donald L. Carcieri, invited all state employees to the Rhode Island State House to kick off his employee wellness initiative, Get Fit, Rhode Island!. State employees heard a series of inspirational addresses by the governor, the president of the University of Rhode Island, the director of health, and other state dignitaries, who spoke about the importance of health and wellness. They outlined the goals of achieving healthier employees, a healthier workplace, and a healthier state. Employees were introduced to the governor's 25 volunteer employee wellness champions (one per state department), who were appointed to facilitate program activities at their

> If your actions inspire others to dream more, learn more, do more, and become more, you are a leader.
>
> *John Quincy Adams*

respective agencies. Each champion came up to the podium to accept a champion shirt embossed with the new Get Fit, Rhode Island! logo. The governor and first lady, Suzanne Carcieri, then led everyone in a ceremonious walk around the statehouse to launch the initiative. After the walk, the governor and first lady socialized and participated in photo opportunities with the wellness champions to build closer relationships with them. The governor inspired his army of leaders of the wellness initiative, provided public recognition, and bonded with his troops.

Although an initiative might not require so many champions, senior leaders still need to provide inspiration and guidance, regardless of the size of the initiative. For example, a school principal may demonstrate support by holding an assembly to kick off a wellness initiative and introduce the school's four wellness champions.

What do we mean when we talk about the importance of senior-level support? Such support goes beyond a leader simply saying, "wellness is important," sending out an e-mail announcement, or allocating a big budget. As with any effort, the leader must continuously engage and inspire employees for success.

Following are 10 of the most effective actions that leaders can take to support wellness programs in worksite, community, and school settings. Any senior leader, whether a governor, mayor, town manager, school district superintendent, school principal, corporate CEO, or store manager, will benefit the wellness initiative by taking these actions.

1. Appoint wellness champions. By appointing champions, leaders imbue the position with status, which increases the commitment of the champions and enhances the public perception of their role. Leaders may appoint champions publicly or send formal invitations to employees to apply.

2. Publicly kick off the wellness initiative at a celebratory launch at the main location and at satellite locations by on-site senior managers.

3. Participate in programs (at least four per year) with participants.

4. Discuss personal wellness experiences and practices with participants.

5. Reward and publicly recognize champions for their efforts at special engagements or through the use of incentives.

6. Provide recognition for participants who have adopted healthier lifestyles.

7. Meet with the wellness director on a quarterly basis for an update and to keep a pulse on the program.

8. Make wellness a priority at meetings with senior-level as well as midlevel managers to ensure top-down support.

9. Put policies in place that support a healthier environment.

10. Continuously inspire troops to deliver the wellness mission.

The wellness director has to make these actions easy for the leader by doing the legwork: planning recognition celebrations for champions and employees, crafting sample e-mails, prioritizing programs for leader participation, and planning programs to fit the leader's schedule. Preparing a calendar of annual events for the leader is helpful for planning and securing leadership participation. If you are appointed to serve as a wellness director, but do not have senior-level support and engagement, make an appointment to discuss the preceding actions with the senior leader.

Meeting With Decision Makers

How do you get an appointment to discuss your wellness initiative with the CEO, senior leader, or decision maker? What do you present? What should the "ask" be to promote your wellness initiative?

- Do your homework! Develop a solid, one-page executive summary of your proposed initiative along with a two- to four-page complete proposal with details. Have a plan, and keep it simple and concise.

- Determine what the "ask" is going to be. What do you need? Be specific in your requests. Keep meeting requests minimal.

- Make an appointment to talk to the senior leader's or decision maker's assistant first. Be courteous to the assistant. Deliver your proposal to the assistant, and ask for five minutes to present your initiative to the senior leader with a focus on short- and long-term employer savings. By asking for only five minutes, you have a greater chance of getting an appointment. Once you have captured the senior leader's attention, you have a greater probability of getting more time or at least a follow-up meeting.

- Be prepared with a tight agenda. Stay on point.

- Make sure your timing is right. Are there competing priorities? Is the organization currently undergoing layoffs or significant changes in leadership? This could make the timing of your proposal good or bad. Talk to others familiar with your proposal to get their input, and use your best judgment about whether to move forward at this time.

- Prepare an "elevator speech," a 30-second synopsis of the benefits of your proposal.

Wellness Director

At a mid-sized university, wellness is a part of the campus culture for students, as well as faculty and staff. Their wellness director has a passion for wellness; his charismatic personality and enthusiasm has spread a wellness movement across the campus like a wildfire. His energy has been instrumental in engaging employees in wellness programs, and his expertise has resulted in high-impact programs that produce results. The director's enthusiasm is what gets employees engaged initially. His knowledge

> Enthusiasm is the yeast that raises the dough.
>
> *Paul J. Meyer*

and strategic abilities are essential for the planning and delivery of targeted, high-impact programs that have kept employees engaged and achieving their health and wellness goals.

This wellness director is described as likeable. He has the ability to get people to work collaboratively and to volunteer their time, expertise, and resources for the initiative. He is the spokesperson for wellness across campus. He is highly visible. Everyone knows the director and the university's wellness mission. What makes this director a perfect choice is the combination of characteristics he possesses. His high energy is coupled with strategic and content knowledge—a powerful combination of personality traits and talents!

The selection of an effective wellness director requires more than just reviewing resumes for qualifications. Certain essential qualities, including personality characteristics, will mean the difference between a mediocre and a targeted, highly successful initiative. Here are 10 qualities that are essential in a wellness director.

1. **Charisma and enthusiasm.** Getting people to change their health behaviors is a difficult task. It requires a wellness director who is personable, passionate, and can enthusiastically sell health behavior change. Collins and Porras (1977) identified two common qualities in leaders that can "almost single-handedly make things happen in organizations." Those leaders most always possess both vision *and* a charismatic personality. A word to the wise: Never underestimate the power of a cheerleader. A successful wellness cheerleader is key. As Ralph Waldo Emerson said, "Every great and commanding movement in the annals of the world is due to the triumph of enthusiasm. Nothing great was ever achieved without it."

2. **Expertise in strategic thinking.** Strategic thinking is the ability to identify steps needed for achieving long-term goals, mapping out routes, solving problems, and reducing barriers along the way. For example, if participation is low, a strategic wellness director develops solutions to counter the issue.

3. **Being a team builder.** Team builders have leadership qualities that people respect. As a result, people are inspired to follow and work hard for team builders.

4. **Being a team player.** A wellness director must be not only a team leader, but also a team player who is committed to the organization, the leadership, and the team.

5. **Cultural sensitivity (a people person).** A people person sincerely cares about people and is empathetic about the challenges people may be facing in their lives. A people person is compassionate, caring, willing to meet people where they are, and able to lead them to where they want to be. Because wellness directors work with diverse populations, they must be sensitive to the perceived needs, barriers, health beliefs, and values of people of all races, ethnicities, ages, and abilities.

6. **Focused flexibility.** A successful wellness director has focused flexibility, or the ability to focus as well as shift gears. By staying focused on an evidence-based wellness plan and not flirting with catchy wellness trends, a wellness director can achieve goals even while adapting and modifying plans seamlessly and quickly, if needed, based on unforeseen obstacles, barriers, or circumstances.

7. **Qualifications and experience.** A qualified wellness director must possess health field–related credentials and experience to identify and make successful evidence-based programming choices. Experience in developing, implementing, and evaluating wellness programs is essential for success. Because there are many moving pieces to a successful wellness initiative, experience is important to keep all the balls in the air. Experience in marketing, communications, and sales is also a must (see chapter 3 for more details).

8. **Commitment and tenacity.** A wellness director who has an unwavering commitment to the initiative has a can-do attitude. Tenacity is needed for overcoming any hurdles and achieving goals. As John Kotter said, "Leaders establish the vision for

the future and set the strategy for getting there; they cause change. They motivate and inspire others to go in the right direction and they, along with everyone else, sacrifice to get there" (http://thinkexist.com/quotes/john_kotter/).

9. **Effective communication skills and the ability to build relationships.** A wellness director who can communicate and inspire people through verbal, written, and nonverbal communication methods helps build valuable relationships with champions and employees.

10. **Ability to organize and manage.** An organized manager is able to orchestrate all the players and pieces needed for making a wellness initiative come together. Because there are many moving parts, the wellness director must manage them all in an organized fashion. This ability is particularly critical in a large organization with multiple sites or satellite locations.

Wellness Champions

A human resources employee of a large national corporation, charged to launch an employee wellness initiative, truly believed in the concept of appointing wellness champions. He believed it was an essential step to ensuring success. However, his plan was to appoint champions later, after the initiative was up and running. This large organization, with multiple offices around the country, was about to launch a full-scale wellness initiative without

> Coming together is a beginning.
> Keeping together is progress.
> Working together is success.
>
> *Henry Ford*

first recruiting an army of troops to infiltrate the organization. The human resources representative was to launch the initiative by sending one e-mail announcement from the senior leader, as well as posting information on the organization's Web site.

Although this appears to be an acceptable and typical launching strategy, would a general go to war without an army? Of course not! Neither should one or two people attempt to launch a wellness initiative. WELCOA warns against this type of "lone ranger" approach to launching a full-scale wellness initiative. It has been proven that the most successful initiatives depend on early recruitment of an army of champions to create a culture that reverberates throughout the organization.

Organizations with the most successful wellness programs put a team of wellness champions in place to support announcements and communications prior to developing and launching their programs. Getting an army of champions on board from the start is imperative for maximum engagement, participation, and success. It truly takes an army to develop and launch an effective wellness initiative.

Consider political campaign strategies. Posters and announcements don't reach the people, *people* reach the people! Political candidates set up campaign offices all around the country and look for volunteers to make calls, give out buttons, and go door-to-door to spread their messages throughout the election campaign. They don't just send e-mails. Because people get bombarded with marketing messages, what remains one of the most effective ways to spread a message is word of mouth, human to human. As John Seely Brown said, "Processes don't do work; people do" (www.earthlingcommunication.com/a/inspiration/famous-and-greatest-inspirational-communication-quotes-for-free.php).

Selecting Champions for Your Wellness Initiative

In 2004, Rhode Island's first lady, Suzanne Carcieri, suggested the use of the word "champion" to identify ambassadors to represent the governor's wellness initiative. She worked with a committee to establish criteria for selecting champions: they should be enthusiastic, passionate, likeable employees who could bring other employees together and motivate them to participate in wellness programs within their respective departments.

In schools across Rhode Island, wellness committees were formed to champion the wellness effort in schools.

Success is more assured when representatives are identified to champion a wellness initiative. If no one has direct responsibility or ownership, things do not get done.

Appointing champions right from the inception of a wellness initiative has a number of benefits:

• **Sense of ownership.** When people get involved in any organizational initiative from the beginning, they become part of the process, they develop a sense of ownership, and they are more committed to its success.

• **Multidisciplinary representation.** Multidisciplinary, or comprehensive, representation on an all-star wellness team engages employees from parts of an organization such as human resources, unions, legal departments, senior level management, purchasing, facility maintenance, safety and risk management, faculty, staff, students, or community program and outreach staff. With multidisciplinary representation, cross-cultural and geographical differences may be considered in developing, tailoring, and implementing the wellness initiative to minimize barriers to, and maximize facilitators for, the wellness program.

• **Division to conquer.** Dividing up the workload among champions at the onset of the initiative will not only help spread the message of wellness throughout the organization to increase participation, but also assist with conquering the workload.

• **Cheerleading.** Champions planted throughout the organization serve as cheerleaders encouraging other employees to participate both at the onset and throughout the course of the initiative.

• **Team players become team leaders.** Champions not only lead their wellness teams within their respective departments, but also serve as team players as members of the organization's champion team.

• **Relationship building.** By leading their wellness teams and serving as a member of the organization's champion team, champions build relationships within their departments and throughout their organization.

Recognizing and Bonding With Your Champions

Recognizing champions is important, particularly if the role does not provide financial compensation. Recognition may come in the form of an award, certificate, small token, or social gathering. In a small setting such as a community-based nonprofit organization, leadership may recognize wellness champions by holding a recognition dinner party. In a larger setting, senior leadership, along with middle management, may demonstrate senior leader support by publicly presenting certificates in front of the entire organization.

The wellness champions also need to bond as a cohesive team. They must have opportunities to get to know each other and to share their expertise. When people get to know the members of their team, they recognize each other's talents and work and begin to support one another, which enhances team loyalty. They will go the distance for their team if they know and respect each other. They are in the game together to win.

Rick Fitzgerald, a senior administrator who championed the highly successful wellness initiative for Rhode Island's Department of Labor and Training as a part of Get Fit, Rhode Island!, once told me: "I began this initiative championing this effort because I was asked by my director, as a response from a request from the governor. But, as time went on, I became more and more committed. I was giving it my all for you and my teammates. I did not want to let my team down!" A solid team is required to accomplish great results. This is not an easy task; it takes constant cultivation. However, when the right people come together and bond as a team (such as the Get Fit, Rhode Island! champion team), greatness may be accomplished collectively!

Team champion meetings should occur monthly. In-person meetings are preferable, but conference calls may be held if they are logistically more convenient or if in-person meetings are not possible. Monthly meetings help accomplish three very important things:

1. They keep the initiative moving forward by keeping the team focused on its mission and goals.
2. They resolve issues that may arise as a group.
3. They keep the team in sync and cohesively bonded.

The following are some suggestions for productive champion meetings:

- Pick a consistent day and time of the month to meet (e.g., the third Tuesday of the month at 9:00 a.m.) that is convenient for all champions.
- Pick a convenient, central location with ample parking for meetings.
- Prepare a yearly calendar of recurring meetings and distribute it to champions.
- Prior to each meeting, forward the agenda to each organizational leader or department head in which the champion is employed to decrease any potential resistance or barriers to attendance that champions may experience.
- Following each meeting, distribute meeting minutes, including a list of attendees, to both champions and organizational leaders or department heads. This keeps leaders informed so they can recognize and support the progress of their champions while also increasing the accountability of both the champion and leader related to the wellness initiative.
- Keep on point during meetings. Stay on agenda items. Do not digress.

Advisory Board or Steering Committee

In 2005, the Rhode Island's state wellness steering committee, a governing body overseeing the state's wellness initiative, met monthly. The first lady of Rhode Island, who had a health education background and a personal interest in wellness, cochaired the Worksite Wellness Steering Committee along with the director of the Department of Health. Members of the committee included myself as director of Get Fit, Rhode Island!, a wellness champion representing the group of state departments, the president of URI, senior-level human resources representatives, union leaders, the state health care insurer, as well as others, including private sector representatives. This high-level committee reviewed group aggregate health insurance claims data as well as other information and data to identify high risks and high health care costs, set the strategic direction of the initiative, solved barriers for the wellness director and wellness champions, and ensured available resources. The steering committee's charge was to plan the long-term direction and monitor the progress of the initiative.

In contrast, a small company might organize a diverse committee of advisors consisting of the CEO, the human resources director, a representative from its health insurance provider, other vendors, and staff members from departments throughout the company such as communications and facilities and maintenance. Whether you are part of a large organization with a statewide infrastructure, a small local company, or community-based organization or school, garnering the support of your community partners (e.g., local colleges and universities, nonprofit organizations, state and local departments of health) will assist in the success of your comprehensive wellness initiative.

A Culture of Health and Wellness

Experts in wellness and health promotion agree that a strong culture of health and wellness is essential to engage and move a population toward successful health behavior change. A healthy environment, healthy policies, senior-level engagement, social support, and sufficient wellness resources must exist for a wellness initiative to not only survive, but also thrive. In addition, effective communication must exist.

Dr. Dee Edington, health promotion expert and author of *Zero Trends* (2009), stated that an organization's culture or environment is the single most important driving force behind successful organizational wellness programs and health behavior change. Dr. Edington has created the following five fundamental pillars for building a successful culture of health and wellness:

1. Senior leadership: Create the vision.
   - Commit to a healthy culture
   - Connect the vision to the business strategy
   - Engage all levels of leadership in the vision
2. Operations leadership: Align the organization with the vision.
   - Brand health management strategies
   - Integrate policies into health culture
   - Engage everyone

3. Self-leadership: Create winners by inspiring individuals to self-manage their health.
   - Help employees not get worse
   - Help healthy people stay healthy
   - Provide improvement maintenance strategies
4. Rewarding behavior: Reinforce the culture of health.
   - Reward champions
   - Set incentives for healthy choices
   - Reinforce at every touch point
5. Quality assurance: Allow outcomes to drive the strategy.
   - Integrate all resources
   - Measure outcomes
   - Make it sustainable

The five-pillar strategy is designed to (1) drive the vision from the senior and strategic leadership level; (2) create a supportive environment via the operations leadership; (3) formulate the objectives through employee self-leadership; (4) reward and encourage positive actions that promote health management; and (5) provide quality assurance measures to assess and improve the success of the effort.

As a health and productivity consultant, I look for the five pillars, IDEAS, and the three Vs when I evaluate an organization's culture of health and wellness.

- **Visual.** Health and wellness must be visible throughout an organization. Health events, in which the senior leaders are visibly present, should be held regularly. Other visual signs of a culture of wellness may include walking paths, bicycle racks, stairwells with piped-in music and pictures to encourage use, hand sanitizers and signage for proper hand-washing technique in the washrooms, health-related posters, senior executives engaging in healthy behaviors, and on-site fitness centers.

- **Verbal.** A verbal dialog on health and wellness must be present throughout the organization. In an organization with a strong culture of wellness, people, including senior leadership, regularly talk about wellness. This may include verbal exchanges on what types of physical activities people enjoy, discussions of healthy recipes, and healthy cafeteria choices. *ACSM* confirms that verbal communication is essential to service businesses, especially health promotion, that rely heavily on personal intention (Cox, 2003).

- **Visceral.** Health and wellness must be deeply woven into the fabric of an organization and everyone in it. Wellness should be part of an organization's mission statement. Organizational policies such as time off for employees who participate in programs, along with an environment and culture that supports healthy behaviors must coincide with a strong individual commitment of members to achieve or maintain healthy lifestyles.

Many of the programs in part II will assist you in incorporating the three Vs into your organization's culture.

Step 2: Data—Collecting Data or Information

How do I measure the ROI of our wellness initiative? How can I tell if our wellness initiative is cost-effective? How do I know whether the wellness initiative is successful? These are a few of the most frequently asked measurement questions posed by senior leaders of organizations that have invested in or have contemplated the implementation of a wellness initiative. These are very reasonable questions and concerns. Senior leaders want to know how to determine whether their investment in wellness will provide financial returns. The answer lies in the data. To measure ROI, you must begin by collecting baseline data on the population, or the members of your organization, and monitor data measures periodically to assess progress. (This is discussed in more detail in Step 5: Success on page 40.)

To ensure that any investment is profitable, you must first collect baseline data for evaluation. Without collecting baseline data from a variety of related sources, or without taking the time to carefully evaluate that data initially and throughout the course of your wellness initiative, you will not be able to discover whether your initiative is making a positive impact. So, what type of data can you collect to measure the success of your wellness initiative? The following data collection strategies— health interest surveys, health risk surveys or health risk questionnaires, and biometric screenings—provide basic best-practice assessments for a comprehensive wellness initiative.

Other Data Sources

Other data sources to obtain baseline health information prior to implementing a wellness initiative include the following:

- Medical insurance claims
- Pharmaceutical claims
- Workers' compensation claims
- Absenteeism
- Productivity
- Job satisfaction surveys
- Stress surveys

Health Interest Survey

The Wellness Council of America recommends the distribution of a health interest survey as an effective initial data collection strategy. A simple, short, nonintrusive survey listing potential programs to be offered as part of a comprehensive wellness initiative helps gauge the interest of potential participants. This information can provide very valuable data to use in the development of a targeted strategic plan also. It is important to know what individuals *need* to improve their health, but knowing what they *want* will allow you attain the highest level of engagement and participation in your programs.

A sample health and wellness survey is presented on pages 29-30. You may customize or tailor this survey to your organization by adding, deleting, or modifying questions. You may distribute the survey in paper form or post it online for completion at computer workstations. If you want help creating a survey from scratch, the Web site Survey Monkey offers "a revolutionary tool to create and publish custom surveys in minutes, and then view results graphically and in real time" (www.surveymonkey.com/).

Sample Health Interest Survey

By taking a moment to complete this brief, anonymous survey, you will help us create health and wellness programs that would be of most interest to you. Should you have any questions regarding this survey, please contact [insert contact person and contact information]. Please place your completed survey in the envelope provided and insert it into the slotted box labeled "Completed Health Interest Surveys" in the mailroom. Your participation is greatly appreciated.

Age:_____   Gender (circle):   M / F

Department or location [if large organization]: _____

Which of the following wellness programs would you be interested in participating in? (Check all that apply.)

❑ Aerobic exercise   ❑ Running clubs

❑ Back care   ❑ Smoking cessation

❑ Cancer screening   ❑ Stretching classes

❑ Cooking classes   ❑ Walking clubs

❑ Coping with stress   ❑ Weight management

❑ Dance classes   ❑ Weight training

❑ Ergonomics   ❑ Yoga and meditation

❑ First aid training   ❑ Other (please list):

❑ Martial arts

❑ Massage   _____

❑ Nutrition   _____

❑ Outdoor sports (e.g., hiking,   _____
   kayaking)
                                       _____

What factors have prevented you from participating in wellness programs in the past? (Check all that apply.)

❑ Financial cost   ❑ Other (please list):

❑ Lack of energy   _____

❑ Lack of interest   _____

❑ Lack of time   _____

❑ Not convenient   _____

>> continued

Sample Health Interest Survey   >> *continued*

How often are you able to attend on-site wellness programs? (Check all that apply.)

❑ A one-time only lecture, presentation, or workshop

❑ Once per week

❑ Twice per week

❑ Three times per week

❑ Daily

What time of the day would you most likely participate? (Check all that apply.)

❑ After work hours

❑ Before work hours

❑ During breaks

❑ During lunch

What day(s) of the week would you most likely participate? (Check all that apply.)

❑ Monday

❑ Tuesday

❑ Wednesday

❑ Thursday

❑ Friday

❑ Saturday

❑ Sunday

What incentives would encourage you to participate in wellness programs? (Check all that apply.)

❑ No incentives needed

❑ Cash

❑ Gift cards or gift certificates

❑ Health insurance discounts

❑ Organizational policy allowing participation during work hours

❑ Raffles

❑ Other (please list):

_____

_____

_____

_____

Would you be willing to pay to participate in a program?

❑ Yes (if yes, please indicate the maximum amount you would be willing to spend per program: $_____)

❑ No

Thank you very much for your input!

From A. Ludovici-Connolly, 2010, *Winning health promotion strategies* (Champaign, IL: Human Kinetics).

A health interest survey is a powerful strategy for introducing a wellness initiative and engaging potential participants. Organizations have reported that people are somewhat suspicious when health *risk* surveys are used as the first data collection tool in the design of a comprehensive wellness initiative. They may question why the organization is requesting sensitive lifestyle information as well as what they are planning to do with this information. By distributing the health *interest* survey first, many organizations report that employees express fewer concerns, and that they are more likely to participate in a health risk survey later. By first asking people what they *want* via the health interest survey, you can then engage them in addressing what they *need* through the results of a health risk survey or questionnaire.

Health Risk Questionnaire (HRQ)

I Took Charge of My Health! This slogan was printed on custom-made stickers given to employees to put on their lapels once they completed their HRQ as part of the launching of a wellness initiative. The purpose of these stickers (which make the program *visual,* an example of the three Vs) is similar to the *I voted* stickers people wear after voting to promote others to do the same. The stickers create a buzz by encouraging others in the organization to attend the event, complete the HRQ, and start taking charge of their health!

Administering the HRQ is an essential step in determining the health risk behaviors of a population. A model HRQ asks questions that evaluate health risks as well as people's readiness to change their health behaviors. They are available from most health care providers, state and local public health departments, and private wellness vendors.

Tip

Following are several sources for health risk questionnaires:

- University of Michigan (www.hmrc.kines.umich.edu/hra/info.cgi?demo=1 &username=webhra-)
- State or local health departments
- Health insurance providers

The HRQ is typically administered on an annual basis, providing valuable health information on a population over time (i.e., health related trends). It is a key tool for evaluating wellness program outcomes or progress. As such, the HRQ should be a scientifically reliable and validated instrument. Non-technically speaking, a reliable questionnaire is one that would give the same results if you used it repeatedly with the same population or group. For example, a reliable questionnaire will give the same results on Tuesday as it did the previous Monday. A validated questionnaire is one that has been shown to measure what it purports to measure. A reliable and validated HRQ can be used in pre- and post-evaluations of wellness initiatives, as well as in the evaluation of short- and long-term trends over time. A reliable and validated HRQ should be developed by, or in consultation with, someone with expertise in program evaluation or statistics to ensure that the results are meaningful.

The process of simply administering the HRQ may be considered a part of a health intervention because it is designed to raise individual health awareness via self-assessment. The HRQ also provides an organization with valuable information on the health of its population for effective wellness program planning. The administration of the HRQ should always be followed with a wellness program or implementing a health intervention based on the results.

ACSM's Worksite Health Promotion Manual (Cox, 2003, pg. 47) cautions: "Many health promotion practitioners have made the mistake of investing too much of their resources in a HRA (Health Risk Assessment) or HRQ. While an HRQ is a very important component, without the necessary resources for diligent follow-up, program success will not be achieved. A HRA alone will not create behavior change."

Sample questions on an HRQ may be related to the following:

- Lifestyle behaviors such as diet, exercise, smoking, and seat belt use
- Preventive health care (e.g., annual physical exams, routine checkups)
- Stress and mental illness
- Readiness to change lifestyle behaviors

Suggestions and Considerations for Administering the HRQ

Suggestions

- Plan an event. Designate an entire day during which people can come and take the HRQ, get their biometric screenings (discussed later), pick up some health information, and get inspired to take charge of their health! Offer refreshments and set the stage to attract people to stop by and participate (see chapter 3).
- If offering an online assessment, open a computer lab or set up laptops or kiosks where people may come and get help completing the assessment. This reduces a barrier for those who may not be computer savvy.
- If administering a paper version of the HRQ, provide an empty envelope that participants can seal before they submit their completed HRQs. This will ease concerns around confidentiality or protecting the privacy of personal health information (see Considerations).

Considerations

- Choose an HRQ that is scientifically reliable and validated
- The HRQ should be compliant with all current, health-related state, federal, and other government or federation regulations such as the Health Insurance Portability and Accountability Act (HIPAA) (www.hhs.gov/ocr/privacy/); the Americans with Disabilities Act (ADA) (www.ada.gov/); and the Genetic Information Nondiscrimination Act (GINA) (www.genome.gov/24519851).
- Should you offer an online or paper assessment? This would depend on the number and the geographic location of employees or groups, access to computers, and resources for distribution and data collection. Paper assessments require more resources and are more labor intensive.

- The HRQ should measure health risks as well as people's readiness to change behaviors (see chapter 3).
- For maximum participation in assessment completion, offer immediate incentives (e.g., raffle entries, gift certificates, health-related giveaways).
- Offer the HRQ for a limited or defined time period such as two to three weeks. Offering the HRQ for an open or longer period could lead to procrastination and nonparticipation (see chapter 3).
- Use the data from the HRQ to develop the strategic plan for your wellness initiative or program(s) to maximize impact.
- Avoid providing large incentives for HRQs as they consist of self-reported data collection measures

Biometric Screenings

A man once told a nurse who was providing blood pressure screenings at an on-site biometric screening worksite event, "If I knew my blood pressure was so high, I would have filled the prescription for my blood pressure medication that my physician gave me at my physical six months ago." These were stunning words from a man whose blood pressure was through the roof! His blood pressure numbers were well over normal values. In fact, they were in such a dangerous range that the nurse requested that the man immediately call his physician, who saw the man in his office that very afternoon. The nurse later stated that if this man had not attended the screening event and seen his physician immediately, there would have been a high probability that he would have had a serious cardiac event. In other words, this screening event may, indeed, have saved his life.

Biometric screening events provide detailed assessments of basic health indicators, including blood pressure, body mass index (calculated from height and weight), cholesterol (HDL and LDL), and blood glucose. Such events are very valuable for creating awareness and providing educational opportunities for participants in worksite, community, and school settings. It is advantageous to offer biometric screenings in conjunction with the HRQ. Participants can then more accurately answer questions on the HRQ versus relying on estimates of their personal health data.

Suggestions for Administering Biometric Screenings

- If you cannot offer a full array of biometric screenings, because participants may not have a lot of time to participate at one time, offer one or two screenings at a time over the course of several days. For example, offer blood pressure screenings one day and body mass index measurements another day.
- Offer multiple opportunities for biometric screenings during the launch of the HRQ for the most accurate responses on the HRQ.

Step 3: Evaluation—Evaluating Data, Setting Goals, and Developing a Strategic Work Plan

As a health and productivity consultant, I have observed organizations collect a wealth of baseline data from the variety of sources mentioned earlier. While observing, I do not mindfully evaluate the results or use them to create a well-crafted operating plan. I begin my work with them by evaluating data, setting goals, and developing targeted strategic plans. It is important to take time to sift through the data to accurately depict the health status and health behaviors of your organization to develop an appropriate strategy for improvement.

After collecting data (step 2), is it critical to spend time examining and evaluating the information. The information can reveal the focus for your initiative, as well as specific, population-based programming needs. Review dietary information, exercise patterns, smoking prevalence, general health indicators from the biometric screenings, and the prevalence of acute and chronic illnesses or diseases. After data evaluation and reflection, you are ready to set SMART goals (see Setting Goals) and establish a written strategic plan based on factual data.

Evaluating Data

After reviewing all of the data collected from the health interest survey, the HRQ, and biometric screenings, organization leaders decided to focus on weight loss for their employees. Prior to looking at the data, the administration was considering launching a smoking cessation program. However, the data indicated that few employees were smokers, and the smokers generally indicated they were not ready or interested in quitting at that time. However, the data showed a high prevalence of obesity and interest and readiness to reduce weight. The wellness director and senior leadership were clear about the need to focus on high-risk behaviors that most employees were concerned about and ready to change first.

Setting Goals

Thomas Carlyle said, "A man without a goal is like a ship without a rudder." An organization without goals is subject to every shift in direction. If you want to stay on course and reach your port of destination, you must set goals. Wellness initiative goals are like any other goals. To set effective goals, you must think SMART. SMART goals are as follows:

- **Specific.** A goal should not be general, but include specific details. A specific goal must answer questions such as what do you want to achieve, and it should define specific objectives or processes for exactly how you intend to achieve it.
- **Measurable.** Establish specific forms of measurement criteria to evaluate success. When you measure your progress, you are more likely to stay on track and achieve your goals. Suzanne Carcieri, the first lady of Rhode Island, once referenced a popular quote, "If you don't measure, you don't care." Another popular saying with many variations is "you can't manage what you don't measure."

- **A**ttainable. A goal may be challenging for an organization, but it must be attainable.

- **R**ealistic. A realistic goal matches the resources, energy, and desire to achieve the goal within the specified time frame (see the next point).

- **T**ime sensitive. Set your goals with a timetable; do not have an open-ended time frame.

So how do you set SMART goals? Here is an example:

The members of an employee wellness committee evaluated all of their available data to determine their wellness goals. They examined the results of their health interest survey and their HRQ, as well as the previous year's health insurance claims data. They discovered that 20 percent of their employees were using tobacco. The HRQ revealed that 15 percent of them were contemplating quitting. Employees were on the right track to improving their health. As a result, the committee set a goal of reducing the number of tobacco users from 20 to 10 percent in year 1. Defined, specific objectives included offering 100 percent of tobacco users nicotine replacement therapy and evidence-based, smoking cessation intervention.

This goal is SMART. It is *specific* (reduce number of smokers by 10 percent); it is *measurable* (they could measure tobacco use rates before and after the program); it is *attainable* (many people reported a desire to change this behavior in the HRQ); it is *realistic* (they had an effective, evidence-based tobacco cessation program ready to implement); and it is *time sensitive* (a one-year program).

Many organizations fail to set specific outcome goals, yet expect outcomes. Be sure to set SMART goals, and just as important, be sure to monitor progress often to adjust your strategy as needed to achieve your goals.

Developing a Strategic Work Plan

Once you set SMART goals, it is important to craft a written plan outlining how you intend to achieve them. The strategic, or operating, plan provides direction, focus, and alignment for the initiative. Once the plan is developed, it serves as the continual guiding and reference document to keep the initiative on track. Share it with senior leadership, wellness committees, and champions to ensure that everyone is on the same page and moving in the same direction.

> A goal without a plan is just a wish.
>
> *Larry Elder*

The Wellness Council of America (WELCOA) identified the following seven components of an exceptional strategic plan:

1. A vision or mission statement for the wellness program that incorporates the organization's core philosophies

2. Specific goals and measurable objectives that are linked to the organization's strategic priorities

3. Time lines for implementation

4. Roles and responsibilities for completing objectives

5. An itemized budget sufficient to carry out the wellness plan
6. Appropriate marketing strategies to promote the wellness plan
7. Evaluation procedures to measure the stated goals and objectives

Jean Kapetanios, a regional wellness director for UnitedHealthcare, assists many large organizations with their wellness initiatives. Jean assisted with the development of the strategic plan used to guide the direction of Get Fit, Rhode Island! Once we developed our individualized plan, we referred to the plan at each monthly meeting of our wellness champions, continually refining it to meet population-based health needs. As the director of Get Fit, Rhode Island!, I referred to the plan on a weekly basis to ensure that we were keeping on track, staying focused, and planning ahead. The agenda of our monthly meetings was driven by that particular month's wellness program as part of the overall initiative or strategic work plan. This allowed us to keep moving toward our goals and prevented us from veering off course. Our plan was the rudder of our ship, keeping us from blowing around in the wind and never reaching our destination. For progress, one must have a data-driven work plan and use it to stay on course!

Step 4: AEI Programming—Developing, Implementing, and Evaluating Awareness, Education, and Intervention Programs

AEI programming encompasses the following three programming categories:

Awareness

Education

Intervention

Research has demonstrated that more than 80 percent of individuals are **not** ready to take action and change their health behaviors at one given time (Prochaska, Norcross, DiClemente, 2006). With this in mind, Awareness, Education, and Intervention programs represent three categories of programming designed to appeal to a wide variety of participants and those who are at different levels of preparedness for behavior change. Most wellness programs fall into these three categories, and all three program types are covered in part II.

Awareness programs do just as the name implies. They increase participant awareness of the importance and benefits of healthy lifestyle behaviors and the risks associated with unhealthy lifestyle behaviors. Awareness programs also prepare participants for more extensive programs. These programs can also serve as reminders. One may be as simple as a stairwell sign encouraging people to take the stairs instead of the elevator. As a general rule, awareness programs are not intended for, nor effective at, creating behavior change. However, they may increase readiness for more extensive behavior change interventions. Awareness programs are especially effective at moving contemplators to a preparation or action stage of behavior change (Cox, 2003).

Education programs teach participants how to practice healthy lifestyle behaviors, but they do not actively engage participants in behavior change (e.g., a lecture, presentation, or workshop on preventing heart disease). Participants in the contemplation or preparation stage can move closer to the action stage through education programs.

Interventions are multifaceted programs that are typically offered over a longer period (e.g., 8 to 12 weeks). Interventions provide participants with opportunities for behavior change, as well as opportunities to increase their awareness of and knowledge about the behavior(s) that the intervention is targeting (e.g., nutrition, physical activity, preventive health care). Interventions are the most effective type of programs for health behavior change but typically attract individuals in the "action" stage of readiness.

Dr. Michael Cryer, national medical director for Hewitt Associates, describes the three types of programming as a three-legged stool. All three legs are necessary to keep the stool balanced. All levels of programs have their place and their benefits. The three types of programs also appeal to people at different stages of change, as described in chapter 3, and help make wellness more visible in the organization. A balance of AEI programming is necessary for increased participation, engagement, and success.

Programming Strategies

American Idol, a top-rated television show for many years, masterfully engaged people to not only tune in to view, but also participate in the decision-making process by calling in their votes. We may apply some of these techniques to health promotion and wellness in order to engage participants in wellness programs.

- Involve people in the process. People respond well when they are involved in the process as well as the outcome. Use every opportunity to engage people in program selection, promotion, and evaluation. Administer group interest surveys, conduct focus groups, and promote Internet blogs.

- Supplement the content of the main program with complementary programs.

- Keep programs time sensitive. Like American Idol, try running programs for a limited time rather than all year long as a way to keep excitement levels high. Limit programs to 8 to 12 weeks. People tend to remain engaged when they see an end in sight or are aware that a program has a limited time offering. However, continue to support and promote program efforts for the target behaviors throughout the year to solidify positive health behavior changes. It is a delicate balance between keeping programs fresh and exciting, and running them long enough to result in positive health behaviors. A health or clinical consultant, or subject matter expert, can help you tailor that balance to your specific population and goals.

- Focus on two or three targeted health behaviors for a longer period of time to increase your chance of success. This will allow time for your population or target audience to progress through the stages of change to create successful results and outcomes on the behaviors. Remember that sometimes less is more. This is

>> continued

particularly important with a limited budget. If you have limited funds and you attempt to spread your budget thin by addressing too many target behaviors, you may be throwing seeds in the ocean. You may never see an impact and your investment will be washed away.

- Set a time line. The following is a sample time line for wellness programs:
  - **January to March:** Weight management
  - **April to June:** Physical activity
  - **July to September:** Farmers market (fresh fruits and vegetables)
  - **October to November:** Stress management
  - **December:** Smoking cessation

Awareness Programs

"After two weeks of seeing *Take the Stairs* signs at elevator entrances and on the doors of the stairwells on the way to the elevator, I finally decided to take the stairs to the second floor, and only take the elevator for three floors instead of five," declared an employee of a children's hospital. Simple health behavior prompts may get people to improve their daily habits. Another example of an effective visual prompt is the American Lung Association's black lung display to increase awareness of the dangers of smoking.

The following are two types of awareness programs:

- **Prompting healthy behaviors.** By pointing out health behavior alternatives or choices, prompts such as stairwell posters and healthy choice signs in the cafeteria or on vending machines may prompt healthy behaviors by raising awareness.

- **Reminding of the pros and cons of healthy behaviors.** If, in addition to encouraging people to take the stairs, a stairwell poster highlights the health benefits of taking the stairs versus taking the elevator, it also serves as an educational tool.

"Exercise has been shown to reduce the mortality rate from heart disease in half and can significantly reduce the rate of obesity. Come in and sign up today to reduce your health risks." This radio advertisement for a health club provides a sound bite, increases awareness, educates listeners, and may get some people to act. Through the power of suggestion and in an age of information, awareness programs may be very effective. Because many people report knowing the reasons they should or should not engage in certain health behaviors, full-scale education programs may not always be necessary. People may benefit from simply being reminded of healthy alternatives. Awareness programs may be very successful at engaging people who may not yet be ready or prepared to change their health behaviors. After prolonged exposure, they may become more likely to want to take steps to improve their health behaviors (see chapter 3). Reminder systems—such as postcards, brochures, or e-mails—can also be effective at preventing relapse and promoting maintenance of health behaviors (Cox, 2003).

Education Programs

Education programs teach people about specific health topics. They can be as simple as promotional materials, newsletters, or table tents, or may provide more extensive content in the form of lectures, presentations, or workshops that include practical, or hands-on, techniques. For example, the state of Ohio hosted a healthy heart event for its citizens. Cardiologists provided educational presentations on ways to prevent and treat heart disease, and representatives from the American Heart Association distributed brochures and resources to attendees.

Intervention Programs

Intervention programs are typically 8 to 12 weeks long because this is the minimal length of time needed for behavior change. Intervention programs do work! After participating in the Just Move It physical activity program for eight consecutive weeks, for example, one participant reported doubling the amount of time she spent doing physical activity each week.

Which Type of Program Is Most Recommended?

The decision of whether to provide an awareness, education, or intervention program depends on a variety of factors, although a balance of each type is recommended:

- Interests, needs, and readiness to change of the target population determined by data collection and evaluation
- Organizational environment
- Vision, mission, and goals of the organization
- Budget or available resources
- Capacity to offer a balance of all three types of programs

Here are some additional suggestions to keep in mind for programming:

- Ensure that programs complement and do not compete with each other. If you offer multiple programs targeting one or more health behaviors, ensure that they are complementary. To maximize participation and program effectiveness, consider offering one primary evidence-based intervention and supplement or augment that with an awareness or education program on the same topic.
- Consider issues relevant to your organization, current culture, and climate. The state of Delaware's wellness program, DelaWell, offered a series of financial and stress management programs at the time the state was about to institute a series of layoffs. DelaWell offered state employees programs relevant to their current needs and interests.

>> continued

Which Type of Program Is Most Recommended?   >> *continued*

- Be sure programs are what participants want (i.e., based on results of health interest surveys) as well as need (i.e., based on HRQ and claims data). At the University of Rhode Island, results of a health interest survey of facilities and maintenance staff revealed an interest in healthy cooking and easy recipes. We were surprised to learn that these primarily male employees often prepared the family dinner because they were the first to arrive home from early work shifts. As a result, we offered a nutrition program focused on healthy, easy-to-make dinner recipes and it was a hit!

- Consider the season or time of year. Some programs are better received at certain times of the year. For example, people may be more interested in stress management in the fall or winter during the holidays when they tend to be more stressed and less active outdoors. Spring is a good time to offer physical activity, and summer is a good time to offer nutrition programs as there is an abundance of fresh fruits and vegetables.

- Ensure programs comply with all current health-related state, federal, and other government or federation regulations such as the Health Insurance Portability and Accountability Act (HIPAA) (www.hhs.gov/ocr/privacy/); the Americans with Disabilities Act (ADA) (www.ada.gov/); and the Genetic Information Nondiscrimination Act (GINA) (www.genome.gov/24519851).

- Consult with legal council on proper medical screening and waivers for participation in wellness programs.

Step 5: Success—Measuring, Monitoring, and Reporting Your Successes and Lessons Learned

To determine whether your initiative has been successful, you should use the data assessment tools mentioned earlier in this chapter pre- and postprogram implementation and year after year. This way you can monitor any change in key health indicators in your population over time. These measurements should mirror the data collection efforts discussed in step 2 and will generally be quantitative; that is, describing or measuring *quantity* (e.g., the number of smokers in the population, the percentage of employees on workers' compensation, the reduction in specific medical claims). Process, or descriptive, measures, which are more qualitative, may be collected throughout the duration of your wellness initiative. These focus on the *quality* of your initiative (e.g., program satisfaction surveys). (See page 41 for a sample program satisfaction survey.) These types of surveys also capture important data such as the number of participants at each wellness program, which may be used for tracking attendance. After you have examined short- and long-term data trends, you can reevaluate your initiative, report on successful outcomes, and make adjustments to your programming efforts, such as updating or revising your wellness goals and strategies and your strategic work plan as needed.

Sample Program Satisfaction Survey

By taking a moment to complete this brief, anonymous survey, you will help us determine whether [insert name of program] met your needs, interests, and expectations. The information you provide will help us improve or modify future programs. Your input is greatly appreciated.

Please circle the most appropriate response according to the following scale:

1 = Strongly Disagree	4 = Somewhat Agree
2 = Disagree	5 = Strongly Agree
3 = Agree	

1. This program was relevant to my health needs and interests. 1 2 3 4 5
2. The program contact person or instructor was an effective communicator. 1 2 3 4 5
3. The program contact person or instructor was knowledgeable and able to answer questions. 1 2 3 4 5
4. The program met my expectations. 1 2 3 4 5
5. I enjoyed participating in this program. 1 2 3 4 5
6. I would recommend this program to a colleague. 1 2 3 4 5
7. How has this program changed your knowledge, attitudes, skills, beliefs, or behaviors related to your [insert target behaviors of program]?

   _____

   _____

8. What recommendations do you have for improving this program?

   _____

   _____

9. Please indicate how participation in previous wellness programs have helped you in the following areas according to the following scale:

1 = Not Helpful	3 = Helpful
2 = Somewhat Helpful	4 = Very Helpful

Reduced sick visits	1	2	3	4
Reduced emergency room visits	1	2	3	4
Increased preventive care visits	1	2	3	4
Decreased number of days you have been ill	1	2	3	4
Increased productivity	1	2	3	4

Please note any additional comments below:

_____

_____

Thank you very much for your input!

From A. Ludovici-Connolly, 2010, *Winning health promotion strategies* (Champaign, IL: Human Kinetics).

Whether they are outcome or process measures, all measures of your wellness initiative allow you to detect and report on successful outcomes as well as lessons learned that you may use to modify or adapt your overall wellness initiative or individual programs. In this way, you can maximize your success in achieving your goals, which, in turn, will garner more top-down and bottom-up support to improve the health and wellness of the people you are working with.

Cultivating Your Wellness Programs

Developing a successful wellness program is a lot like cultivating, planting, and maintaining a garden. Once you cultivate the soil or lay the foundation for planting the seeds by introducing or kicking off a single program or comprehensive wellness initiative, your work has just begun. You now need to tend your program daily by providing all of the sunlight, water, and other nutrients, or program supports, that it needs to thrive. If you want to increase program participation and promote positive results, you must continually weed your garden or program of all the factors that impair participation and positive results. You may need to tweak your program marketing strategies, deploy other strategies, or allocate additional or different resources as needed. The more consistently you provide the sunlight, water, and other nutrients your program needs, the healthier the fruits of your labor will be.

Summary

Researchers have identified specific foundational components and steps necessary for developing, implementing, and sustaining a successful, comprehensive health promotion initiative. The concepts outlined in this chapter have been developed or endorsed by leaders and organizations in the health promotion industry. The concepts in this chapter are key **IDEAS**:

Infrastructure (building the internal foundation to sustain a wellness initiative)

Data (collecting data or information)

Evaluation (evaluating data, setting goals, and developing a strategic work plan)

AEI programming (developing, implementing, and evaluating awareness, education, and intervention programs)

Success (measuring, monitoring, and reporting your successes and lessons learned)

Building your wellness initiative on a foundation of IDEAS is essential for success within any type of organization or setting.

Creating Engaging
Wellness Initiatives

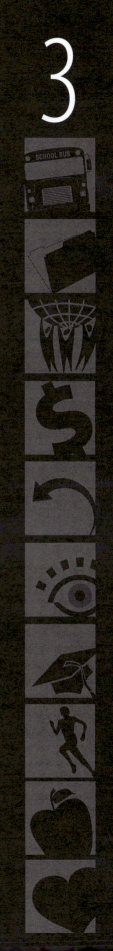

From the moment you open the glossy, enticing travel brochure to the time you enter the stately wrought iron gates, you are attracted. Within a very short period, you become completely engaged and entrenched in the culture you have entered until you exit the resort. The culture may remain a part of you for weeks and, in some cases, months after departure. In my case, it never vacated.

Club Med knows exactly how to attract, engage, and sustain guests' interests and attention all too well. It not only knows how to attract guests by providing a variety of relaxing antidotes, but it also knows how to engage guests in daily physical activity, and on vacation to boot! Everything I learned about motivating people to exercise, I learned at Club Med. I have told this to many diverse audiences at business conferences I have presented at, as well as in many college classes I have taught. Of course, I admit that this statement *is* an exaggeration, but it does hold some merit. And here's why.

Early in my career, I had the pleasure of working for Club Med in the French Caribbean for a short time. I was assigned to a few locations to train guest organizers, or GOs, to teach exercise classes and to assist with setting up on-site fitness centers. Some guests declared that they had not exercised for many years, yet they kept active daily at Club Med. *What is going on here?,* I asked myself. I began to pay attention to what Club Med GOs were doing, and after a few days I got it. I began learning from *their* lead. Here is my story.

When I arrived at Club Med in Guadalupe, I was fresh out of college and a newly certified health fitness instructor. I knew all the proper protocols for delivering individualized, safe, and effective exercise prescriptions. When I got to the location where I was to train the GO, I was horrified! I immediately went to Jerome, the chief of the village, and declared, "This location is unacceptable!" It was on the beach. I was concerned about floor surface, or the lack of it, with steep slopes and uneven surfaces on which someone could easily twist an ankle. I was concerned about the blazing sun of the Caribbean, which could lead to dehydration and sun exposure (skin damage) while exercising. I was concerned about improper footwear because people did not wear shoes, or much else for that matter (a story for another book)! I was concerned . . . .

Before I could verbalize all of my concerns, Jerome cut me off. "Oh, Onnie (Annie)," he pleasantly said in his French accent. "No problem, no problem. Onnie, just have *fun*!" I returned to the beach where my protégé, Pierre, was waiting for me. Pierre was not well versed in English, and I was not well versed in French. So, on top of every other barrier, Pierre and I had a communication barrier! *This just keeps getting better and better!,* I sarcastically said to myself.

Pierre signaled to someone to start the music. It blared from a pair of very large speakers that were perched up high on stands facing the ocean and hidden among the palm trees. I requested that the music be turned down so that guests could hear the instructions while we gathered a crowd. My request was granted. I then walked around the beach and invited everyone to join us. I began the class with about a half dozen people. I was leading the class while showing Pierre how a safe and effective exercise class should be conducted. After a few minutes, Pierre disappeared. Shortly after I noticed his absence, the music volume was turned up again! I looked down the beach and spotted Pierre. He was gathering guests like the pied piper while gyrating to the loud music in his leopard print Speedo. He then proceeded to walk back to the class with a large crowd of people in tow. Beach chairs were emptying as just about everyone was joining in the class, dancing, moving, and laughing. No one was following my instructions. No one could hear them. No one seemed to care. But, everyone was having a blast!

Throughout my time at Club Med, Pierre and I learned how to strike a balance between safe and effective exercise instruction, and entertaining, engaging instruction. He taught me how to meet people where they wanted to be (on the beach) and doing what they wanted to do (moving to their own beat). And, it worked! We adapted to the environment by avoiding lateral movements in the sand, which, in turn, avoided ankle sprains. We taught half the class in the water to address improper footwear and hydration concerns and we gave water breaks. Although it is sometimes difficult to strike a perfect balance between safety and engagement, I learned that it *is* possible. Now, in challenging exercise situations, I just think of Jerome and say to myself, No problem!

I share this story to demonstrate the importance of consciously creating an engaging environment and culture for your wellness programs and avoiding homogenizing wellness. Health promotion should not be delivered like a clinical, sterile program if you expect high engagement. It is not just about the content of your programs and adherence to technical scientific methodology, but how you position them, deliver them, and communicate them. It is about when, where, what, and who. It is about the art and science of developing and delivering engaging wellness programs.

Engaging participants in your program is not easy, and *sustaining* engagement can be even more challenging. You must understand how to build a strong infrastructure based on the IDEAS presented in chapter 2 and have a strong communication and marketing plan. An understanding of individual behavior change theories and strategies is also helpful. If you can orchestrate all of these strategies and launch engaging programs (see part II), you can mobilize large groups and communities to change their health behaviors. This chapter details marketing and behavior change strategies and provides examples that you can implement in any setting to promote program engagement, while having a great time in the process!

Goetzel and colleagues (2001) state that one of the 10 traits of the most successful health and productivity programs is that people have fun in the process (see page 17). Just remember Club Med's approach—*No problem!*

Staging

The delightful smell of freshly popped popcorn permeated the halls of the YMCA. Members followed the trail of the scent and the sound of popping popcorn to find a festive wellness event in progress. Brown University was on site recruiting members for a nutrition intervention called Good for You. Brown staff set up a colorful vintage popcorn cart, decorative tables, and colorful banners bearing the Good for You logo, along with a wide array of props and materials to attract people to the event.

Program staging is the art of setting the stage to entice people to participate in a program or event, and to keep them engaged for an extended period of time. Home staging, or real estate staging, is described as anything that can help home sellers make their homes more attractive and appealing to potential buyers. The home stager does this by adding plants, artwork, furniture, and other attractive accessories to make the space look its best. Staging also involves the proper placement of items for maximum impact and reducing clutter to create a more open, inviting space. A real estate agent once said, "One may think that buyers make logical decisions, but often emotions guide buyers to what just feels right. Creating a warm, inviting, and attractive atmosphere can make a huge difference in the sale of a home."

Staging of wellness programs is based on the same concept. People make decisions to purchase products and services based on emotions, as well as logic. If a program looks appealing, they will be more likely to check out what is going on, and they will stay longer if the environment is appealing. If the program appears uninviting and boring, people are more likely to walk on by.

Successful Staging

The annual health fair at the Community College of Rhode Island (CCRI) is always staged to perfection, and participation shows. As you enter the event, you are greeted by wellness champions and their team members wearing team shirts at the welcome table. The wellness team stands on either side of the welcome table, not behind it, to give a warm welcome and shake hands with guests as they arrive. The welcome table has warm lighting being thrown from lamps, fresh flowers in vases, and colorful balloons along with a variety of beautiful gift baskets that are displayed as raffle prizes and incentives. Live music is provided by students from the music department. Vendors such as UnitedHealthcare display seasonally decorated booths with colorful sand toys such as pails and shovels beside literature on sun protection, providing a punch of color and interest. UnitedHealthcare also provides free sunscreen samples and skin screening with DermaScan, a simple device that uses ultraviolet light to show sun damage that is invisible to the naked human eye. The annual CCRI health fair engages all of the senses!

The college's athletic director and wellness champion, Joe Pavone, launched CCRI's wellness program as part of Get Fit, the governor's state employee wellness initiative. Mary Pecchia, a member of Joe's wellness team, has since taken over CCRI's successful wellness program, and the beat goes on. Each year, the CCRI health fair draws hundreds of faculty, staff, and students. The president of CCRI, Ray Di Pasquale, is an active participant in the annual health fair. President Di Pasquale doesn't just do an obligatory walk-through, but receives all of the health screenings. In addition, he personally welcomes his faculty, staff, and students and demonstrates sincere appreciation for all of the hard work of the members of his wellness team through public recognition. President Di Pasquale emulates senior level support.

To optimally stage a wellness program, you must engage all of the senses—sight, sound, taste, smell, and touch. Following are some suggestions on how to do so.

Sight

- Display your program logo on large banners or posters printed on high-quality paper or cloth and with attractive colors. Include your logo on giveaway items. The more people see your logo, the better chance they will have of recognizing and identifying it.

- Use visual aids such as display boards and display items such as portion-size food samples, plastic arteries with cholesterol or plaque buildup, and so on. Visual aids may add the punch needed for an effective presentation. Visual learning has been found to improve learning by up to 400 percent. Approximately 65 percent of the population consists of visual learners and the human brain processes visuals 60,000 times faster than it does text (www.visualteachingalliance.com/). With these facts in mind, more health promotion strategies should include visual components.

- Props may create interest, engage participants, and help sustain participation if they become an ongoing part of your program.

- Use colorful linen tablecloths that are coordinated with the overall color scheme of your display table or booth. Ensure that they are clean and pressed.

- String lights, bright-colored helium balloons, and other decorations attract attention and create a festive atmosphere. String lights may have a theme such as flamingos or palm trees. Mini white lights also are engaging during any season.

- Provide exercise demonstrations.

- Set up television monitors to play health-related DVDs.

- Gift wrap raffle boxes for tickets. Decorate gift baskets for winning raffle tickets.

- Plan your program around a theme. For example, a program with a Hawaiian theme may give away leis or tiki torches (if outside).

- Use table lights, candles (if allowed to burn), or other lighting sources. Florescent lighting is not conducive to creating a warm and inviting atmosphere.

Sound

- Music may be a very motivating component of a wellness program. Have you ever listened to upbeat music upon entering and while browsing through a store? What effect does this have on your mood? Does it make you want to purchase?

- At wellness programs, tabletop or standing floor water fountains may provide soothing and relaxing sounds to attract and engage participants.

Taste

- An effective strategy for attracting and engaging participants is to provide free food and beverage samples. Grocery stores and shops often do this to attract potential customers to new foods and tastes.
- Provide samples of air-popped popcorn with no butter as a healthy snack.
- Set up fresh fruit baskets for participants to choose fruits from.

Smell

- Aromas can be added to the atmosphere by holding cooking demonstrations and making popcorn.
- Aromatherapy (e.g., candles, oils, and potpourri) is another way of attracting participants through smell.
- Flowers and fragrant plants in baskets provide a welcoming visual as well as fragrant aromas.

Touch

- Provide hands-on demonstrations as part of your health screening programs (e.g., plastic replicas of arteries with cholesterol or plaque buildup).
- Have some of your wellness program staff available in front of welcome and display tables to shake hands and greet participants.
- Provide on-site chair massage.

Tips for Staging

It is important to prepare a staging plan, as well as provide ongoing reminders of your wellness initiative or programs. The following tips can help:

Preparing a Staging Plan

- Engage your wellness team or committee in the process. Make use of everyone's creativity and talents.
- Review your resources. Ask vendors (if applicable) to stage their booths.
- Discuss the selection of a theme for your program such as a Hawaiian luau, a particular holiday, or a seasonal theme (e.g., summer, winter, spring, or fall).

Between Wellness Programs

- Keep wellness on the forefront on a daily basis.
- Create a wellness corner, area, or center by securing a physical presence in each facility. Include an information center with stocked brochure racks along with postings of all upcoming wellness programs.
- Maintain a wellness bulletin board. Change information on a regular basis.
- Select programs in part II (such as An Apple a Day).

Social Marketing and the Four Ps

On any given day of the week, if you watch television, you will be inundated with an incredible amount of fast food and fatty food commercials. We are the targets of aggressive marketing campaigns that promote unhealthy and large meals whether we are hungry or not. David Katz, MD, MPH, director of the Yale-Griffin Prevention Research Center and a renowned expert in nutrition, weight control, and public health, agrees with the fact that we, along with our children, are bombarded with commercials promoting unhealthy foods and beverages. At the Third Annual Obesity Congress in Washington, DC, Dr. Katz said to the audience, "I don't know about you, but I think I will remember to eat even if I'm not reminded to."

Advertisers work hard to encourage us to consume fast food high in saturated fat, cholesterol, sugar, and sodium and low in vitamins, minerals, and fiber. In fact, we are encouraged to consume larger portions of fast food with discounts on "value meals." However, Dr. Katz noted that "value meals" actually cost more than smaller portion sizes. Although advertisers promote spending less to get more unhealthy food, consumers spend twice as much trying to lose the weight they gained while saving money! Because two-thirds of Americans are now overweight or obese, weight loss has become a billion-dollar industry in the United States.

To slow or reverse the obesity epidemic (a top priority of the World Health Organization and many state and national campaigns), we need to fight back with equally effective messages for healthy behaviors. Marketing has a huge impact on consumer behavior, on what we choose to do and choose not to do. We may not even be conscious of the many influences that marketing has on our daily choices. Sometimes we may not even realize why we are drawn to a store or to a product. The effects may be subliminal. The good news is that we can use enticing marketing strategies to attract people to wellness. Social marketing assists us in this process.

Social Marketing

One well-known definition of social marketing is "the application of commercial marketing technologies to the analysis, planning, execution, and evaluation of programs designed to influence voluntary behavior of target audiences in order to improve their personal welfare and that of society (Andreasen, 1995, page 7.)

> The importance of applying social marketing principles to the development of social policy and strategy cannot be overstated, especially in the area of health.
>
> *Alan Andreasen, professor of marketing,*
> *Georgetown University*

Philip Kotler and Gerald Zaltman conceptualized social marketing as a discipline in the 1970s. They realized that the marketing principles that were being used to sell products to consumers could be used to sell ideas, attitudes, and behaviors. Kotler and Zaltman describe social marketing as "differing from other areas of marketing only with respect to the objectives of the marketer and his or her organization." Social marketing seeks to influence social behaviors that benefit the target audience and the general society, not the marketer (www.social-marketing.com/Whatis.html). "Like commercial marketing, the primary focus is on the consumer—on learning what people want and need rather than trying to persuade them to buy what we happen to be producing. Marketing talks to the consumer, not about the product" (www.social-marketing.com/Whatis.html).

According to both the U.S. Centers for Disease Control and Prevention (CDC) and the American College of Sports Medicine, social marketing consists of effective, evidence-based techniques that increase engagement and promote positive behavior change by

- using commercial marketing strategies;
- influencing voluntary (not coerced) behavior change (not just increased awareness or increased knowledge); and
- promoting the goal of improved personal and societal welfare.

Tip

The CDC has developed a comprehensive CD-ROM-based social marketing tool, CDCynergy, available at www.orau.gov/cdcynergy/soc2web/default.htm.

Social marketing incorporates the same concepts as commercial marketing. Important marketing concepts include the following (www.social-marketing.org/sm.html):

- The ultimate objective of marketing is to influence action.
- Action is undertaken whenever target audiences believe that the benefits they receive will be greater than the barriers they face or costs they incur.
- Programs to influence action will be more effective if they are based on an understanding of the target audience's own perceptions of the proposed engagement.
- Target audiences are seldom uniform in their perceptions or likely responses to marketing efforts and so should be partitioned into segments.
- Marketing efforts must incorporate all of the four Ps (described next).
- Recommended behaviors always have competition, which must be understood and addressed.
- The marketplace is constantly changing, and so program effects must be regularly monitored and management must be prepared to rapidly alter strategies and tactics.

The Four Ps of Marketing

There are four strategies to consider when planning intervention activities for reaching a target audience from multiple perspectives: Product, Promotion, Place, and Price.

These are collectively known as the four Ps of marketing, and all four components are instrumental in considering how to design a social marketing campaign.

- Product: Who, what, why, when
- Promotion: Marketing, advertising, and selling wellness programs
- Place: Where wellness programs will be available and how they will be distributed
- Price: How much the wellness program(s) will cost

Product

To engage people, programs have to be enticing. Product relates to who, what, why, and when. When considering the *who* in product delivery, you must take into account both who is delivering the product and to whom the product is being delivered.

Who Is Delivering the Product? If you are not knowledgeable about your product, or wellness program, and if your presentation is not engaging, consumers will likely not attend. Adrienne Evans, senior health insurance analyst for Rhode Island's health commissioner, refuses to book health educators to perform wellness programs if they deliver information by PowerPoint presentations. "No PowerPoints," Adrienne declared to her program vendor when booking a stress management program series. Adrienne knows that her employees find PowerPoint presentations boring and would quickly lose interest.

Adrienne is the wellness champion for the state Department of Business Regulation, where they average 80 percent program participation. Yes, 80 percent. Adrienne has been able to achieve this outstanding percentage *without* incentives. Adrienne offers targeted, engaging interventions based on concrete data. She also screens her presenters to ensure that the products they are delivering are not only steeped in scientific evidence, but also interactive and fun.

Adrienne knows her employees, and she knows what will attract them to wellness programs and captivate their attention. Superior program delivery, along with superior senior-level support by the department's director, Michael Marques, ensures the success of their wellness programs. The result is great wellness product delivery by people who know how to engage their audience.

To Whom Is the Product Being Delivered? It is of utmost importance to consider your target population throughout all phases of the design, implementation, and evaluation of your wellness initiatives or program to ensure that you are reaching those at highest risk of chronic disease. Healthy People 2010, the prevention agenda of the U.S. Department of Health and Human Service (HHS), is designed to achieve two overarching goals: (1) increase quality and years of healthy life and (2) eliminate health disparities. The second goal of Healthy People 2010, to eliminate health disparities, includes differences that occur by gender, race or ethnicity, education or income, disability, geographic location, and sexual orientation (www.healthypeople.gov/). This important demographic and socioeconomic data may be collected as a routine part of your health interest survey, health risk survey or HRQ, as well as biometric screening (see chapter 2).

As racial and ethnic minority groups become an increasingly larger proportion of the U.S. population, the future health of the country will depend on effectively engaging diverse populations in our wellness initiatives and programs and reducing their risk of chronic disease. "The future health of the nation will be determined to a large extent by how effectively we work with communities to reduce and eliminate health disparities between non-minority and minority populations experiencing disproportionate burdens of disease, disability, and premature death" (Guiding Principle for Improving Minority Health, www.cdc.gov/omhd/about/disparities.htm).

According to the U.S. Centers for Disease Control and Prevention's Office of Minority Health & Health Disparities (www.cdc.gov/omhd/amh/dbrf.htm), Americans who are members of racial and ethnic minority groups, including African Americans, American Indians and Alaska Natives, Asian Americans, Hispanics, and other Pacific Islanders, are more likely than whites to have poor health and to die prematurely. Culturally appropriate wellness initiatives and programs, based on evidence-based prevention research that identifies the causes of these disparities and reduces potential or perceived barriers, are critical for successfully eliminating health disparities by gender, race or ethnicity, education or income, disability, geographic location, age, and sexual orientation.

What Is Being Delivered?   As organizations struggle with improving program participation, the need to employ both evidence-based methods related to program content and behavior change theories is becoming increasingly clear. To maximize program engagement and participation, be sure that the methods you use to design, deliver, and evaluate your wellness programs are evidence based, or grounded in scientific research, as well as based on the behavior change theories presented later in this chapter. For example, Active Living, a program offered by Human Kinetics, is based on the findings of Project Active, a research study conducted by the Cooper Institute in Dallas, Texas. This groundbreaking program not only is steeped in proven programmatic methods, but also weaves in behavior change research to maximize engagement and results.

Why Are You Delivering the Product?   Before you can begin a wellness program, you need to ask yourself why the program is needed. For example, after reaching a staggering 90 percent participation rate in its HRQ (chapter 2), Hewitt Associates felt confident about what type of programs its associates most needed. The *why* was answered by the results of the data. Relying heavily on communication through technology, Hewitt Associates works with worldwide clients. Because employees at Hewitt Associates spend a great deal of their workdays in front of computers, it was not surprising to find that associates needed to increase their physical activity. This organization used the results of its HRQ to deploy a social networking physical activity program steeped in behavior change theories. Hewitt Associates answered the *why* before making the decision to design and deliver a wellness program.

When Are You Delivering the Product?   When making the decision to offer a specific program, think about when to offer it, including the time of year, day(s) of the week,

Product Tips

- Offer products or wellness programs that people both want and need based on the data you collected (i.e., from health interest surveys, health risk questionnaires, and biometric screenings). See chapter 2 for more information.

- Make your product attractive to your audience.

- Ensure that your product or wellness program was created based on scientific research using validated outcome measures. Don't reinvent the wheel.

- Offer a "fully baked" program that has been pilot tested on a small audience to work out all the bugs.

- For maximum engagement and participation, make your program *fun*!

- Report on effective, measurable outcomes and lessons learned.

- Offer a mixture of online and visual programs on site. Remember that you are trying to build a culture of wellness. Your audience must see programs and people in action.

and time of day. *When* influences engagement. Remember, timing is everything. For example, over one-quarter of employees at a worksite attended the Stress-Less Day program held in mid-December. Employees reported a high level of stress during the holiday season. If this program had been offered another time of year such as the summer, attendance may have not been so high.

Promotion

Promotion involves marketing, advertising, and selling wellness programs. Promote wellness and health improvement opportunities with creativity and through a variety of channels and strategies that will maximize engagement. Advertising, public relations, sales, and entertainment may all be used in promotion strategies. Integrating a variety of promotional strategies is most effective. Discovering what product or wellness program is most appealing to your audience will help you develop a targeted promotional plan. Focus groups, surveys, or both, may also provide this information.

The goal of a promotional plan is to create and sustain demand for your wellness program. Paid advertising and brochures are one way to promote a health and wellness program; there are other methods as well. Consider creating a brand and logo, holding wellness events, writing educational editorials, developing a program Web site, setting up program displays, and attracting participants to a program. A successful promotional plan integrates all five steps to building a successful wellness initiative (see the discussion of IDEAS in chapter 2) to engage populations in adopting healthy behaviors.

Michelin Tires: Choose Well-Live Well

Michelin Tires is an organization committed to the health and welfare of its employees. Michelin has taken a holistic approach to the company's health care challenges and has introduced a new wellness initiative, Choose Well-Live Well, which goes beyond generic wellness announcements and simply shifting increasing costs of health care to employees; instead, it includes a focus on health from every angle. Michelin has made employee health a top business priority. Michelin's communication experts teamed up with Hewitt Associates to design and launch a comprehensive communication initiative to effectively deliver health and wellness messages prior to introducing Choose Well-Live Well to Michelin employees. Their communication strategies, implemented over time, used the following channels:

- **Brand and logo.** Michelin created a brand and designed an action-oriented logo that fit the organization.

- **Focus groups.** Michelin conducted focus groups with employees and their spouses or significant others to obtain a clear understanding of why employees choose certain lifestyle behaviors. The results of these focus groups shed light on the concepts and beliefs that were barriers to employees being responsible for their personal health. The focus groups revealed that convenience (making healthy behaviors easier and more accessible) and incentives would help eliminate barriers to participation in wellness programs. Michelin then focused on those two areas.

- **Newsletter series.** As part of Choose Well-Live Well, four newsletters were mailed directly to employees' homes. The newsletters offered a more personalized, self-directed tone that encouraged employees to take an active role in their personal health and the health of their loved ones.

- **Drive Time.** A clever addition to the Choose Well-Live Well communication strategies was an estimated completion time for each wellness activity. To keep within the transportation industry theme, Michelin added a clearly visible bubble labeled "Drive Time" to all internal communication documents requiring a response or action. This gave employees an upfront estimate of the amount of time it would take to complete requested surveys, questionnaires, or other programs. For example, the "Drive Time" to complete the HRQ was 15 minutes. This was a highly effective way to get people to carve out the time needed for participating. If participants don't know the time commitment, they may anticipate a greater time investment than required, they may procrastinate, or they may not participate at all. This is especially true in our time-conscious society in which people have increased workloads and work hours.

- **Incentives.** A multifaceted incentive strategy was developed to reward employees for completing each wellness program as part of the overall Choose Well-Live Well wellness initiative.

Anita Doncaster, a senior manager and head of the communication practice for Hewitt Associates, worked with Michelin for several years. Anita emphasized that a key component of Michelin's success was strong senior leadership support. "The best communication strategy could not have engaged as many employees in the program if senior leadership was not fully on board with the initiative," Anita remarked. Michelin's vice president of benefits was fully supportive of and engaged in Choose Well-Live Well every step of the way.

An example of effective promotion involves a marketing firm in Manhattan that was retained to create a social marketing campaign for the Great American Smokeout. One of the promotional strategies they used involved an old ice cream truck. Go figure! This marketing firm sent an ice cream truck up and down Wall Street with music to spark public interest and messages on the benefits of quitting smoking painted on the outside of the truck. They distributed information on the many health benefits of living a smoke-free life and traded packs of cigarettes for cups of coffee. Brilliant! Executives from up and down Wall Street came out to see what the buzz was about.

A creative strategy such as this engages people in behavior change. Long gone are the boring, long-winded lectures on the risks associated with unhealthy lifestyle behaviors. Remember Adrienne's declaration of no PowerPoints? Make your wellness program fun and engaging. Think outside of the box.

The more touch points and strategies you can deliver to potential participants in wellness programs, the better chance you have to penetrate the multitude of messages people are exposed to on a daily basis. Multiple delivery methods include mail, e-mail, voice mail, brochures, posters, and social networking. Repetition of multimessaging approaches is also critical. If you have the resources, hire a consulting or marketing company to assist with your communication needs. If communication expertise is available in your organization, be sure to capitalize on it. Get creative. Get out of the box to fight this war to create a healthier global community!

In addition to having good marketing and advertising strategies, a wellness program personality or spokesperson can enhance engagement. A variety of corporations have put their CEOs out there as poster children for their products. From Lee Iacocca of Chrysler decades ago, to the new CEO of Sprint, many effective campaigns have featured personalities in their advertising to engage the public. An effective spokesperson or personality matches the product or service that is being marketed and could be a charismatic wellness director (see chapter 2). He or she can inspire and move people toward product, service, or program adoption and, ultimately, brand loyalty.

Rajiv Kumar is the program personality behind Shape Up RI (www.shapeupri.org). Rajiv is also the founder and chairman of Shape Up RI, a very successful series of team-based healthy lifestyle competitions to increase physical activity and reach personal and team exercise or weight-loss goals in Rhode Island. This program is offered to all residents of the state. Rajiv's face is on every e-mail Shape Up RI sends out. He makes many public appearances, and he is present at all of the program's launching and educational events. Participants in Shape Up RI identify with Rajiv. He is a live person, not just a program, and people identify with people.

Rajiv is known as one of Rhode Island's celebrities. As a board member of Shape Up RI, I had a business lunch meeting with Rajiv one day in a small restaurant in the city of Providence. While we were discussing the program, a member of Shape Up RI came up to Rajiv to show him that he was proudly wearing the program's well-known blue wristband. Rajiv, in turn, showed the man that he was wearing his as well. The wristband provided to each participant in Shape Up RI has a twofold purpose. First, it serves as a daily reminder of the commitment participants have made to the program. It is also a way for members to identify and connect with other members of the program, as in this situation. This gentleman went on to thank Rajiv for offering the program and told him of the impact it had made on his life while sharing the impressive fitness goals he was able to achieve. He was thrilled to talk with Rajiv, whose very presence inspires people.

Promotion Tips

- Develop a logo and trademark.
- Have multiple touch points and repetition. The more people who see your wellness program or hear your message, the greater the chance of infiltration. Use multiple delivery methods such as e-mail, voice mail, brochures, posters, table tents, and newsletters.
- Change signage and messaging regularly so they continue to attract attention and do not become invisible.
- Print attractive promotional materials on quality paper of various colors and sizes.
- Ensure that handmade posters are not cluttered with too much information. It is important to research effective techniques if you are designing your own communication materials.
- Retain communication specialists for top-quality results.
- Coordinate messages among your wellness programs, and be consistent with your messages.
- Remember that timing is critical. Promotion should not be for too short or too long a period of time.
- Messages sent about two weeks in advance are remembered better than those sent two months in advance.
- Print or create large posters or banners to place on building entrances one week prior to the launch of your program.
- Leave reminder flyers on your program at employee workstations the evening before it is scheduled to start.
- Create a sense of urgency about enrollment in your program (e.g., limited time, limited space). Offer data collection such as the HRQ within eight weeks prior to the start of your program as opposed to ongoing access.

Selling the program is often overlooked; and its importance, minimized. We often don't think of wellness and sales as related. However, if we are to engage people in adopting healthy lifestyle behaviors, we must sell the benefits of doing so. It just makes sense! "Keep your enthusiasm," Governor Carcieri advised me.

As chief executive officer of Cookson America and joint managing director of Cookson Group Worldwide, he was a businessman prior to serving as governor. He told me about a book on sales that he read early in his career. It stressed the fundamental key to successful sales: enthusiasm. The governor recognized that to engage employees in wellness, we had to sell wellness. And, to sell anything, whether it is a product, a service, a program, or a lifestyle change, we needed to exude enthusiasm and passion about what we were selling. Brilliant! At that moment, I was reminded of the power of sales in health promotion.

Sales Tips

- The most successful salespeople believe in what they are selling. They walk the talk and live a healthy lifestyle themselves. If you don't practice what you preach, people will disregard your product or message.

- Be passionate and enthusiastic about your product. Your enthusiasm will then inspire others to learn more about what you are selling.

- Learn or brush up on sales skills. Attend seminars on sales, read sales books, listen to sales CDs, or take a class in marketing.

- Know your product. Keep up-to-date in the field of wellness to optimize sales and ensure that your delivery is engaging.

- According to ACSM, personal interaction and verbal communication are particularly important when selling a service such as health promotion.

Place

Place refers to where a wellness program takes place and how it is disseminated. Location, location, location! Many are familiar with this popular phrase that applies not just to real estate sales but to adopting healthy lifestyle behaviors as well. Industry consultant Mike Chaet notes that 80 percent of a health club's members live within a 6- to 8-minute drive from the club (http://cms.ihrsa.org/index.cfm?fuseaction=Page.view Page&pageId=15146&nodeID=15). Health clubs, as well as wellness programs, need to be convenient and in close proximity to work or home if people are going to join and utilize the memberships and programs. People are more likely to talk themselves out of participation if the location is not appealing or convenient. To ensure maximum participation, offer programs in places that appeal to the audience and take into account their current lifestyles. Remember the Club Med beach story?

The State of Delaware's wellness initiative, Dela*WELL*, schedules programs in central locations for state employees around the state to maximize engagement and to increase program accessibility by participants. Program location has a big impact on participation. One university offered a farmers market for the campus community at one end of the campus. After finding that participation was low, they moved the market to the center of campus, and participation increased dramatically.

Price

How much should your wellness program cost? When considering price, you must take into account both the financial and nonfinancial costs to participants.

Place Tips

- Chose convenient, central locations with adequate parking whenever possible.
- Make sure the location is appealing with adequate space and lighting. Make sure your location is at a comfortable temperature.
- If you plan to conduct sensitive health screenings, ensure that the visible location also has the privacy to accommodate them.
- Prior to booking a location, survey your potential audience for the most popular choice(s).
- Rotate locations.
- Go to the source. Provide programs at each building if an organization has multiple buildings.
- Ensure that your program has good visibility. Visibility increases exposure, which increases engagement.
- Bring your program to your audience using fitness vans equipped for your needs.

Financial Cost   Prior to designing and launching a program, you must consider the financial cost, if any, to the people you hope to serve. It is important to know up front how much participants would be willing to pay for a wellness program. You may gather this information as part of your health interest survey discussed in chapter 2. If your program is not affordable, cost will be a major barrier to participation. Early in the planning stage, consider all the costs associated with design, implementation, evaluation, and reporting of results. Costs may include materials, personnel and consulting fees, media and communications, rental space, and so on. The programs in part II of this book are ranked as low, medium, and high cost to help you select programs that fit your budget. With senior-level support, program costs may be covered by the organization, split between the organization and its participants, or costs may be reimbursed to participants upon completing a program or achieving their goals.

Nonfinancial Cost   A member of my health club once told me, "I would like to exercise after work more days of the week, but I would be giving up our family dinner, and I am not willing to do that." In this situation, giving up the family dinner would be the price this member would have to pay for exercising more frequently. In social marketing, the price of participating in a program is not only what people may be required to pay monetarily, but also what they would be required to sacrifice for participation. Frequently, the nonmonetary sacrifice is more of a barrier than the financial cost of a program. The price one might have to pay may include missing out on other activities, giving up a favorite habit, not indulging in favorite food choices, and cutting into family time or just discretionary time in general.

The problem is that many people perceive the price of practicing a healthy lifestyle as costly in their time-deprived lives. In a time of extended work and workweeks, and when two or more household incomes are often necessary to make ends meet, people are reporting to be starved for time. When discretionary time is limited, the price of participating in wellness programs may be perceived as too high. As promoters of health and wellness, we often find ourselves competing with the conflicting priorities of the audiences we are trying to engage. However, research has proven that participants are more likely to make time to participate in programs that are fun. People are more likely to take time for things they *want* to do versus making time to do things they *should* do. Part II of this book offers many fun and short duration programs to address this perceived barrier.

We can help potential participant weigh the benefits and costs, or the pros and cons, of participating in wellness programs. One way is to keep promotional materials short and concise so people don't have to spend too much time reading them. It may also be helpful to provide a cost–benefit analysis or statement to demonstrate the value of engaging in programs. This especially holds true when trying to engage senior-level support in an organization. The following section gives you solutions and strategies to address any perceived barriers.

Understanding Health Behavior Change

As a member of the International Health, Racquet and Sportsclub Association's (IHRSA) Health Care Task Force, I presented on a panel at IHRSA's European Congress in Rome in 2005 and in Paris in 2007. David Pickering, chair of the task force, led the panel, titled "Leveraging the Health Care Crisis: Re-engineering Your Thinking to Improve Your Profits." Our presentation drew a large international audience of fitness and wellness professionals. At this European Congress, it became evident that countries around the globe are looking for health behavior change solutions and strategies to assist their clients in adopting healthy lifestyle behaviors. Globally, industry leaders are looking at health behavior change as a plausible aid to assist in the escalating health care costs associated with chronic diseases.

I presented on the successes and lessons learned from implementing a wellness initiative in a statewide government setting and the practical applications of behavior change theories. "How do you change behavior?," was a common question from the audience. I challenged those who were serious about effectively changing lifestyle behaviors to research and take a deeper look into behavior change theories, to learn them inside and out, and to learn how to interpret them and to apply them to health promotion and wellness programs.

James O. Prochaska, PhD, along with several other world-renowned researchers, created evidence-based behavior change models based on interventions to improve a broad spectrum of health behaviors. As practitioners, we and, most important, our audiences would benefit from applying these models of behavior change theories to the design, implementation, and evaluation of our wellness programs.

In my work as a national consultant on employee health and productivity for Hewitt Associates and a scholar in residence at the University of Rhode Island's Cancer Prevention Research Center (home of the transtheoretical model), I have found that many health insurance providers and vendors do not fully understand the true meaning of behavior change, nor how to apply behavior change theories to product design and delivery. Some people will tell you that behavior change is based on effective communication or the drive to obtain incentives that are offered. However, this is not the case. Many of the most well-known behavior change theories presented in this chapter have been proven to improve and sustain healthy lifestyle behaviors through intrinsic motivation.

Once you have attained proficiency in applying these theories to the design and implementation of your wellness programs, your market value will increase as others take note of the success of your programs. Seek out these opportunities. You can be part of the solution and help drive positive health behavior change. Today, we are fortunate to have many tools to assist our clients, employees, and other consumers to move toward a healthy lifestyle.

Abraham Maslow once said, "If the only tool you have is a hammer, then you have to treat everything as if it were a nail" (Prochaska et al., 2006, pg. 88). Dr. Prochaska, a psychologist internationally recognized for his work as a developer of the stage model of behavior change, says, "We have many tools now available in our toolbox to help people make changes" (personal communication). I encourage you to first take a look to see what tools are needed, and then learn how to use them effectively to create a wave of positive health behavior change.

Theories of Behavior Change

If your goal is to change behaviors and sustain behavior change, weaving behavior change theories into the content of your evidence-based programs can help. Marketing and communications assist in engaging participants. However, quality programs—steeped in behavior change theory—are needed for sustaining healthy behavior change. Look at the commercial product industry. Advertising and promotion may initially sell products, but only the quality of the product will result in long-term sales and brand loyalty. This is similar to the difference between engagement and marriage. Communication may lead to engagement, but behavior change results in marriage (sustaining their commitment to long-term wellness). Several models of behavior change are based on the theories presented next.

Transtheoretical Model

The transtheoretical model is based, in part, on five stages related to a person's readiness to change behavior. The five stages of change are precontemplation, contemplation, preparation, action, and maintenance. People are said to progress through these stages at varying rates, and some may vacillate back and forth among the stages a number of times before attaining the ultimate goal of maintenance. The stages of change are better described as spiraling rather than linear. Individuals do not move systematically from one stage of change to the next, and they may not stay at one stage for a long period of time; rather, the way they move through the stage of change may be cyclical (Prochaska, Norcross, and DiClemente, 2006).

The transtheoretical model has shown that people use different processes of change as they move from one stage to another. Application of the model also shows that efficient self-change depends on doing the right thing (processes) at the right time (stages). According to this theory, tailoring health behavior programs or interventions to match a person's readiness to, or stage of, change is essential to successful achievement and maintenance of

Tip

More details on the transtheoretical model are available on the University of Rhode Island's Cancer Prevention Research Center's transtheoretical overview page at www.prochange .com/ttm.

behavior change. For instance, a person who is not yet thinking of stopping smoking (i.e., precontemplation) may be moved toward contemplation through awareness education tailored to her stage; someone who has already stopped smoking (i.e., action) and would like to maintain that behavior change (i.e., maintenance) would require a different form of education or intervention. Programs or interventions tailored to people's specific stages of behavior change have been scientifically proven to be much more effective than a one-size-fits-all approach to changing health behaviors.

How do people move from one stage to another? In general, for people to progress from one stage of change to the next, they need the following (Reprinted, by permission, from Pro-Change Behavior Systems. Available: www.prochange.com/ttm):

- A growing awareness that the advantages (the "pros") of changing outweigh the disadvantages (the "cons")—the transtheoretical model (TTM) calls this *decisional balance.*

- Confidence that they can make and maintain changes in situations that tempt them to return to their old, unhealthy behavior—the TTM calls this *self-efficacy.*

- Strategies that can help them make and maintain change—the TTM calls these *processes of change.* The 10 processes include:

  1. *Consciousness-Raising*—increasing awareness via information, education, and personal feedback about the healthy behavior

  2. *Dramatic Relief*—feeling fear, anxiety, or worry because of the unhealthy behavior, or feeling inspiration and hope when they hear about how people are able to adopt healthy behaviors

  3. *Self-Reevaluation*—realizing that the healthy behavior is an important part of who they are and who they want to be

  4. *Environmental Reevaluation*—realizing how their unhealthy behavior affects others and how they could have more positive effects by changing

  5. *Social Liberation*—realizing that society is more supportive of the healthy behavior

  6. *Self-Liberation*—belief in one's ability to change and making commitments and recommitments to act on that belief

7. *Helping Relationship*—finding people who are supportive of their change
8. *Counter-conditioning*—substituting healthy ways of acting and thinking for unhealthy ways
9. *Reinforcement Management*—increasing the rewards that come from positive behavior and reducing those that come from negative behavior
10. *Stimulus Control*—using reminders and cues that encourage healthy behavior as substitutes for those that encourage unhealthy behavior

Different strategies are most effective at different stages of change. For example, counter-conditioning and stimulus control may really help people in the action and maintenance stages. But these processes are not helpful for someone who is not intending to take action. Consciousness-raising and dramatic relief work better for someone in this stage (precontemplation).

Learning Theory

Start off slowly. Take small steps to progress. How many times have you given this advice to a participant who is sedentary or just starting a fitness regime? This advice is based on a few scientific theories of behavior change. Learning theories postulate that learning a new pattern of behavior, such as changing from a sedentary to an active lifestyle, typically requires modifications of several small behaviors that lead to achieving the target behavior. For example, if an inactive participant sets a goal of exercising for 30 minutes daily, this new pattern may be better adopted and adhered to by breaking down the time into smaller time commitments such as 10 minutes per day. Incremental increases such as adding five minutes each week may assist in permanently shaping a lifestyle behavior to reach a target goal. It must be noted that new patterns of healthy lifestyle behaviors often replace or compete with former patterns of unhealthy behaviors that people often enjoy (e.g., watching television, eating fast food), habitual behaviors (e.g., driving instead of walking short distances), or behaviors cued by the environment (e.g., taking the elevator instead of the stairs).

Often, behavior change is learned and maintained by positive reinforcement and anticipated rewards. Rewards or incentives may include physical benefits (e.g., better health, more energy, improved physical appearance), extrinsic rewards (e.g., receiving praise and encouragement from others, or receiving a small item such as a water bottle), and intrinsic rewards (e.g., experiencing a feeling of accomplishment or gratification from attaining a personal milestone or goal). Intrinsic motivation is motivation that comes from within, whereas external motivation comes from an outside source. Although praise, encouragement, and other extrinsic rewards help people adopt positive lifestyle behaviors, external reinforcement may not result in sustained, long-term change. The most powerful motivator for long-term behavior change is intrinsic motivation.

Self-Efficacy Theory

The basic concept of self-efficacy lies in the center of psychologist Albert Bandura's social cognitive theory. The theory postulates that people are more likely to engage in lifestyle behaviors that they perceive themselves to be competent in or that they have a good chance of succeeding at (Bandura, 1994). Those who believe they can and will perform well are more likely to view a difficult task as something to master rather than something to avoid. If a person does not feel competent or is uncertain about her ability to succeed at or sustain a behavior change, she will most likely avoid it.

Bandura defined self-efficacy as a person's belief in his ability to succeed in specific situations. Bandura's theory postulates that a sense of self-efficacy in a particular situation may play a major role in how a person approaches goals, tasks, and challenges. In the context of behavior change, a person is more likely to attempt and succeed at implementing positive lifestyle changes in areas in which he has a strong sense of self-efficacy.

The following describe the well-documented sources of self-efficacy:

- **Mastering experience.** The more opportunities a person has of succeeding at a task, the more self-efficacy increases. The opposite is also true. Setting small, attainable goals and achieving them is a great way of improving self-efficacy.

- **Social support opportunities.** People with strong and frequent support from social networks are more likely to improve their self-efficacy related to a given task or behavior change. (See the section on social networks next.)

- **Vicarious experience.** You may have heard the expression, "Anything you can do, I can do better." Self-efficacy has been shown to improve by watching someone else succeed at a task. People who witness the success of others sometimes say to themselves, "If they can do it, so can I." Most human behavior is learned observationally through modeling. From observing others, we form ideas on how new behaviors are acquired. These ideas may be used on subsequent occasions as a guide for action.

- **Interpretation of physiological cues.** How a person interprets certain physiological cues such as soreness, fatigue, shortness of breath, satiation, and hunger will affect her self-efficacy related to specific behaviors.

Social Networks and Societal Influences

Research has shown that social networks have a profound influence on behavior change. In a study of a densely interconnected social network of 12,067 people assessed repeatedly over the course of 32 years as part of the Framingham Heart Study, weight gain in one person was significantly associated with weight gain in that person's friends, siblings, spouse, and neighbors. A person's chance of becoming obese increased by 57 percent if he or she had a friend who became obese in a given interval. Among pairs of adult siblings, if one sibling became obese, the chance that the other would become obese increased by 40 percent. Finally, if one spouse became obese, the likelihood that the other spouse would become obese increased by 37 percent (Christakis and Fowler, 2007). This finding demonstrates one example of how social networks may positively or negatively affect health behavior practices or behavior change. Social networking programs, such as Shape Up the Nation (chapter 5), can positively influence behavior change through social networking. The social support (social network) of a team or peers (as opposed to individual programs), and friendly competition can be powerful motivators for sustaining health behavior change.

Researchers have discovered that there are strong societal and cultural forces that affect individuals' health choices and lifestyle behaviors. For example, economic deprivation can foster negative health behaviors (Ulmer, 1984). Furthermore, as many behavior change theories and experts have noted, positive health behaviors are reinforced by social groups and networks. In addition, powerful sociocultural influences and developments, such as the automobile industry, the media (including radio, television, computers, and Internet access), and even fashion have been said to affect lifestyle health behaviors and practices. It is important to recognize the current sociocultural climate in order to completely understand the current influences and relevant determinants of health.

Barriers to Behavior Change

"I know exercise is good for me, but I don't have any time to fit it into my schedule." "I would eat more fresh fruits and vegetables, but they are too expensive." "The classes offered are at inconvenient times for me. I might participate if they were held in the morning." Barriers to achieving health and wellness goals such as these have been well documented (Prochaska et al., 2009). We, as wellness advocates and change agents, would benefit from a better understanding of how to identify barriers to participation by those in our programs, and how to assist them in overcoming them (see the survey on pages 29-30).

Barriers are like sales objections, and overcoming sales objections is a key component of training in successful sales. It has been suggested that a sales objection may simply be a consumer's request for more information. Successful engagement requires helping participants overcome barriers to participation. The more skilled we become at doing that, the more participants will become and stay engaged.

Ten of the most common reasons adults cite for not adopting more physically active lifestyles are as follows (Sallis, Hovell 1990; Sallis et al. 1992).

- Do not have enough time to exercise
- Find it inconvenient to exercise
- Lack self-motivation
- Do not find exercise enjoyable
- Find exercise boring
- Lack confidence in their ability to be physically active (i.e., low self-efficacy)
- Fear being injured or having been injured recently
- Lack self-management skills, such as the ability to set personal goals, monitor progress, or reward progress toward such goals
- Lack encouragement, support, or companionship from family and friends
- Lack of access to parks, sidewalks, bicycle trails, or safe and pleasant walking paths convenient to their homes or offices

Other reported barriers include the following:

- Costly programs (see the earlier section, Price)
- Poor-quality programs (i.e., weak in content or substance, not fun, or both)

- Programs that require the use of technology. Many people proficient at using computers don't enjoy spending leisure time on computers. Those who are not proficient at computer use often report that they find computer use stressful.
- Lack of energy or motivation
- Cultural and language barriers (see the earlier section, To Whom Is the Product Being Delivered?)

Asking potential participants to identify barriers to participation may help you design and implement a successful wellness program. You may gather this information as part of your health interest survey, discussed in chapter 2.

Pros of Behavior Change

You must communicate the pros of exercise, or any health behavior, to counter any perceived barriers. "It is important to note that research has shown that the pros of changing a behavior must go up twice as much as the cons (barriers) decline to result in adoption of a behavior so twice as much emphasis should be placed on increasing the pros than on decreasing the cons" (Prochaska et al., 1994, 39-46). The pros of exercise include the following:

- Improved body image, self-image, and self-esteem
- Increased energy
- Increased metabolism
- Improved heart function
- Increased endorphins
- Improved enjoyment (fun), social enjoyment
- Decreased anxiety and depression
- Decreased body fat
- Decreased cholesterol
- Decreased physical and emotional pain

Role of Incentives

Incentives, such as promotional items, gift cards, cash, health insurance premium reductions, and raffles, provide external motivation. Incentives have proven to increase participation in wellness programs. However, the question of whether incentives permanently change and sustain positive health behaviors remains. Behavior change theories that have proven to be most effective at long-term behavior change focus on intrinsic motivation, or motivation generated from within the person. People may sign up for a wellness program because of an incentive, but they may not sustain the health behavior(s) associated with the program after receiving the incentive. Although incentives have been shown to increase participation, they may not consistently improve outcomes (Pronk, 2009). Nonetheless, as long as evidence-based behavior change theories are embedded in program methodologies, providing incentives is still recommended for initial program engagement. The goal of incentives should be to activate individuals to initially engage in health improvement programs. With that said, to get participants to sustain engagement, it is critical to move them to become intrinsically motivated, increase self-efficacy, and into the action stage of health behavior change. If you can intrinsically motivate participants, you have a greater chance they will sustain the behavior long-term, even if the incentive is removed.

The type and value of incentives vary greatly. Some of the most popular incentives are discounts on health insurance or co-payments, cash, gift cards, raffle tickets, and small giveaway items. One year, a municipality offered a $100 cash credit on each employee's health insurance co-payments as an incentive for completing an online HRQ. The following year, they offered a T-shirt. The city had a greater participation in year 2! Why was this so? Was it the immediate gratification of receiving the T-shirt on site? Was it other variables such as increased comfort level in completing the HRQ, improved promotion of the HRQ or the incentive, or a change in climate or leadership within the organization in year 2? Any or all of these could have been factors. This example shows that we may not always know what motivates people to action. So, even if you don't have a large budget for incentives, little things may go a long way in helping you accomplish your goal. It's all about what your population values (Pronk, 2009). It is important to discover what is important to your population and resist making assumptions on what they value. The needs and interest survey presented on page 41 includes incentive questions that can assist you in determining what is of value to your population.

Based on an investigation of incentives across 124 companies, Michael Taitel, PhD, of Alere, a leading health management services company, advised that the type of incentive does not matter as much as the value of the incentive (Taitel et al., 2008). The type of incentive may be tailored to the unique culture of the company. For example, one of Alere's clients is an engineering company with 188 employees dispersed throughout five locations in three states. The president of the company actively participated in the program and encouraged employees to earn points by completing a wellness assessment, a physical exam, one challenge, one online seminar, and one community event. For incentives, participants were given $50 for completing the HRQ and an additional $250 for earning 21 activity points by a set date. This company's participation rate for the HRQ was 81 percent. After a year the company saw a 23 percent decrease in blood pressure and a 60 percent decrease in dietary fat intake among employees. Furthermore, the percentage of employees in the high-risk health category decreased from 35 percent in 2007 to 28 percent in 2008. The client was very pleased with the results and attributed the success to a well-designed evidence-based behavior change program that offered a health fair in each location at the start of each year, appropriate incentive amounts, regular communication, and visible management support.

Taitel et al. (2008) also found that companies with effective communications and a strong organizational commitment to wellness may achieve high rates of participation with lower-value incentives (see figure 3.1).

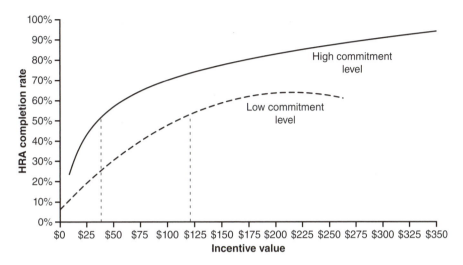

Figure 3.1 Health risk assessment completion rate by incentive value and communication or organizational commitment level.

Adapted, by permission, from M.S. Taitel et al., 2008, "Incentives and other factors associated with employee participation in health risk assessments," *Journal of Occupational and Environmental Medicine* 50(8): 863-872.

Suggested Incentives

- Promotional items (branded with the program logo): T-shirts, water bottles, hats, Frisbees
- Cash
- Raffle items: Fitness equipment such as treadmills, Wii Fit games, gym memberships, healthy cooking classes
- Discounts on health insurance premiums (worksite setting)
- Gift cards: Sporting good stores, health stores or farmers markets, yoga or exercise classes

Suggested Incentive Tips

- Surveys may help identify the type of incentives that appeal to your audience. Questions related to incentives may also be added to your health interest survey or HRQ (see chapter 2).
- Promotional items with the logo of your wellness initiative or program (e.g., coffee mugs, water bottles, note pads) may serve multiple purposes:
  - Low-cost promotional incentives may help promote your initiative or program and increase participation. For example, to participate in a biometric

>> *continued*

Suggested Incentive Tips   >> *continued*

screening offered at the Rhode Island statehouse, we offered each participant a red heart-shaped stress ball. Returning to their offices with their stress balls sparked the interest of other employees. "Where did you get that?" or "What did you have to do to get that?", many asked. Also, many employees kept their stress balls on their desks where they were accessible for use, and where they also served as free, ongoing advertisement for our wellness initiative.

- Low-cost promotional incentives provide immediacy. Immediate incentives reinforce positive behavior at the point of engagement. Immediacy is a recommended incentive strategy (Pronk, 2009).

Summary

This chapter describes the art and science of health promotion engagement. The highest-quality, evidence-based health promotion and wellness programs can, and will, fail if people are not attracted to participate in them. More important, if participation is not sustained over time, adoption of long-term behavior change will not occur. Understanding how to bridge the gap between science and practice is essential to engage participants in wellness programs. The bridge is built with a variety of the attraction, behavior change, creative or artistic, and psychological engagement strategies described in this chapter. This chapter details staging and social marketing, the theories of health behavior change, barriers to behavior change, and the role of incentives in wellness program participation. These strategies are important considerations for the successful design, engagement, implementation, and evaluation of wellness initiatives and programs, such as those presented in part II of this book.

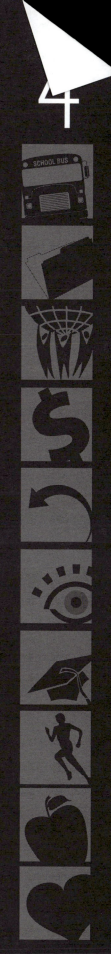

Improving and Expanding Existing Wellness Initiatives

What are the latest strategies in the wellness industry? What are the hot trends? As a national subject matter expert on employee health and productivity for Hewitt Associates, I hear these questions frequently from organizations that either have a wellness initiative in place or are looking to take their wellness programs to the next level. Upon evaluation, these organizations sometimes discover that they are not effectively or completely implementing the five steps to building a successful wellness initiative presented in chapter 2 (i.e., IDEAS).

I once asked the leaders of an organization that was struggling to increase program participation if they had wellness champions to help spread the message of wellness throughout their organization. Although they reported that they did, together we found that their champion network had been inactive for quite some time. We also found little to no senior leadership support for a wellness operating plan that was sitting on a shelf collecting dust.

Before looking at what's hot, you may need to go back to the basics. As Albert Einstein said, "To raise new questions, new possibilities, to regard old questions from a new angle, requires creative imagination and marks real advances in science." Revisiting the basic building blocks of your wellness initiative or program may raise new questions, leading to new possibilities that may be both creative and reflective of the most recent, evidence-based advances in wellness and health promotion. A wellness initiative, whether mature or new, must always be built on a solid foundation to prevent mediocrity or, even worse, collapse. Once you can ensure that you have met all of the basic criteria, or IDEAS, for building a successful wellness initiative presented in chapter 2, you are ready to move on to more advanced steps.

A Solid Foundation

My father owned a construction company for more than 30 years. He was a brilliant, intuitive businessman of great integrity who understood the importance of building and maintaining a solid foundation. He once was contacted by a homeowner who wanted to add a second level to his home. During his evaluation, he found significant cracks and weaknesses in the foundation, which he knew would mean that it would not hold up under the weight of the addition. My father recommended that the foundation be repaired prior to any addition work. The homeowner was not happy in the least and told my father that he wanted to go ahead with the project. My father declined to bid on the addition. The determined homeowner sought a second opinion from another contractor who was willing to do the addition without repairing the foundation. The foundation worsened, and prior to beginning new construction, the home experienced severe leakage in the basement. Furthermore, the town building inspector denied a permit for the new level to be built because of the defects in the foundation. It was not long before the homeowner called my father again, sincerely thanked him for his honesty, and asked him to fix the foundation. My father repaired the foundation and worked for this client for years on many other projects. Through this and many other similar experiences, my father imparted to me many great lessons on the importance of honesty, integrity, and building (anything) on a solid foundation.

Many people do not want to spend time fixing foundations. The work itself is not sexy or cutting edge. Foundations are hidden beneath the surface, cannot be showcased, and are not recognized for their worth. However, a strong foundation is critical to sustaining many things, including wellness initiatives. In the short term, it is often easier and faster to build on what you already have in place, no matter what the condition of the foundation. However, as the foolish man who built his house on sand learned, a successful, long-term outcome requires a solid foundation. Before building additions onto your existing wellness initiative or program, go back to the basics and ensure that your foundation is solid.

To evaluate whether your initiative has successfully met all of the basic criteria for success as outlined in chapters 2 and 3, ask yourself the following questions.

Infrastructure

- Do senior and midlevel leaders actively participate in five or more programs per year, each year?
- Do senior and midlevel leaders keep abreast of the progress of the wellness initiative or program? Are they well versed in the mission of the initiative and its goals to the extent that they are aware of other important organizational initiatives?
- Do senior and midlevel leaders recognize wellness champions on a regular basis?
- Does the wellness director possess the qualities outlined in chapter 2?
- Are wellness champions actively involved and engaged in the initiative? Do they contribute to the team? Do they meet monthly and average 80 percent attendance at meetings?
- Are wellness champions able to tell you what the goals of the initiative are?
- Do wellness champions possess the qualities outlined in chapter 2?
- Does the steering or oversight committee meet regularly to review short- and long-term goals and progress, and minimize barriers to progress?

Data

- Did you offer a health interest survey to your employees? Did you receive at least 50 percent participation?
- Did you offer a health risk survey or health risk questionnaire (HRQ)? Did you receive at least 50 percent participation?
- Did you offer biometric screenings? Did you receive at least 50 percent participation?
- Are your participation numbers increasing over time?

Evaluation

- Did your steering or oversight committee review all the data collected?
- Did you take time to review and discuss findings to set priorities and goals?
- Did you develop a written plan and time line based on the data collected?
- Do you stick to your plan and make adjustments when needed?

AEI Programming

- Are you offering targeted programs based on the results of collected data?
- Are your programs evidence-based or grounded in scientific research?
- Are your programs engaging? Are they fun?
- Are your participation numbers increasing over time?
- Are you offering a balanced blend of awareness, education, and intervention programs?

Success

- Are you addressing the health interests and needs of your audience?
- Are participants satisfied with the program?
- Are you conducting process and outcome evaluations?
- Are you using the results to refine or redefine your programs to maximize success in achieving your goals?

Engagement for Health Behavior Change

- Do you have a plan that addresses the four Ps of marketing?
- Do you have a brand and logo for your initiative?
- Are you reducing reported barriers to improving health behaviors?
- Are you promoting the pros of changing negative health behaviors?
- Are your programs incorporating evidence-based theories of behavior change?

It is important that you answer these questions with brutal honesty and accurately assess your initiative as it stands. In his book *Good to Great*, Jim Collins (2001) notes (quoted material from pages 70-72), "You absolutely cannot make a series of good decisions without first confronting the brutal facts." In his research, the good-to-great companies Collins studies, unlike the comparison companies, "redefined the path to greatness with the brutal facts of reality." I challenge you to take Collins' advice and make an "honest and diligent effort to determine the truth of the situation" prior to strategizing on how to take your program to the next level. Once you evaluate your current wellness initiative with the brutal facts of reality, the right moves and decisions will not only reveal themselves, but they will have a greater effect. In turn, you will achieve a higher level of long-term success.

If you honestly answer "no" or "I don't know" to any of the preceding questions, it is important to go back to the basics to build on or improve your existing foundation before adding the next level. Revisit chapters 2 and 3 to review and strengthen the basic building blocks of your initiative prior to considering more advanced techniques for improvement. Additionally, remember my father's advice regarding the essential requirement for a solid foundation. A solid foundation will ensure maximum participation and positive results. If you answered "yes" to all of the questions, you are ready to take your wellness initiative to the next level!

Taking Your Wellness Initiative to the Next Level

After ensuring that your existing wellness initiative has successfully met all of the basic criteria for success, you can use any of several strategies to take it to the next level. *ACSM's Worksite Health Promotion Manual* (Cox, 2003) has identified the following four areas meriting serious consideration for mature or seasoned initiatives or programs:

Increasing senior-level support

Clock building versus time telling

Developing key organizational health indicators

Broadening the understanding of the actual determinants of health

Increasing Senior-Level Support

According to *ACSM's Worksite Health Promotion Manual* (Cox, 2003, pg. 123), effective wellness initiatives, particularly mature initiatives, require "complete, unwavering support of senior corporate officers." Senior-level support is defined as "more than just a casual interest or management by abdication." With maturity, there is often an urgent need to increase senior-level support and to engage, or to increase the engagement of, midlevel leadership or management for ongoing success.

The ACSM (Cox, 2003) recommends the following key roles of leaders of mature wellness initiatives:

- Communicating the vision
- Providing a positive role model
- Allocating adequate resources and instituting supportive policies
- Recognizing and rewarding employee and champion success

Chapter 2 detailed strategies for increasing the interest and engagement of leadership over time. To take your wellness initiative or program to the next level, ensure comprehensive support from all of your organizational leaders, both senior and midlevel. Leadership's engagement in the wellness policies, programs, and environmental or cultural changes in any type of organization is one of the most important foundational elements for a successful wellness initiative.

David Anderson, PhD, senior vice president and chief health officer of StayWell Health Management and an expert in health promotion research, recommends strengthening the culture of wellness and senior leader support within an organization to foster continual growth of wellness initiatives or programs and to maximize positive health outcomes. The results of a study published by Dr. Anderson and colleagues suggest that a worksite culture supportive of wellness and a comprehensive communications strategy, along with other factors such as incentives, may all play a role in increasing HRQ participation (Seaverson, Grossmeier, Miller, and Anderson, 2009). In this study, a worksite culture score was derived from nine items including verifiable senior and midlevel management support, infrastructural support (i.e., physical environments and policies supportive of wellness), the wellness team, an integrated strategy that is woven into other aspects of health and wellness programs offered within the organization (e.g., disease management, behavioral health, other health benefit programs), and dedicated on-site staff with wellness responsibilities. Organizations that demonstrated a strong culture of wellness experienced greater engagement in their wellness initiatives than those that did not.

Clock Building Versus Time Telling

The ACSM's second recommendation involves the critical step of enlisting many people to join the wellness effort and avoiding the appointment of a single qualified leader. In the book *Built to Last* (1977), authors Collins and Porras described how some organizations have been able to survive and thrive in spite of overwhelming circumstances and a highly competitive business environment. They referenced the organizational concept of clock building versus time telling. Clock building is the long process of melding the various talents and skills of people in a group to build a cohesive, effective team that can thrive far beyond the capabilities of one single leader. To increase stature, influence, and effectiveness, and to survive over time, mature initiatives must be disseminated to a variety of key players throughout the organization. As discussed in chapter 2, it is important to recruit an interdisciplinary army of champions or ambassadors and to continue to develop that army so that wellness infiltrates throughout the organization. Once troops are recruited, leaders must sustain their engagement.

Developing Key Organizational Health Indicators

Mature programs improve and grow through ongoing data collection, evaluation, and appropriate action derived from valid and reliable sources such as health risk appraisals, biometric screenings, health care claims, and reports on absenteeism and workers' compensation. Using these data as "intelligence" to develop and continually refine or redefine a strategic plan will result in sound programming efforts, maximized engagement, and successful outcomes. Successful, mature programs continually seek improved participation in their health interest surveys, health risk surveys or HRQs, and biometric screenings, year after year.

Get Fit, Rhode Island! has taken their program to the next level by continuing to review and refine their strategy to target the top medical and pharmaceutical cost drivers specific to their population. Get Fit, Rhode Island! most recently implemented a "Rewards for Wellness" incentive strategy to enhance engagement and target key health behaviors. As a result, Get Fit, Rhode Island! has significantly increased program engagement and has begun to assess cost savings via medical claims data.

Aaron B. Schrader, MS, health promotion coordinator for the state of Delaware's comprehensive wellness program, Dela*WELL*, believes that "successful long-term wellness programming is a dynamic, rather than static process that advances based on employees' changing interests, thoughts and health concerns" (personal communication). Schrader has found that conducting regular needs assessments and evaluation techniques allows for the stratification of risks and the development of ongoing programs or events (i.e., health seminars, campaigns, or wellness challenges) that target employees' unhealthy lifestyle behaviors and ultimately promote positive change. This assessment process has involved online and paper-based Health Risk Assessments (HRA) with subsequent projection of annual avoidable health care costs based on aggregate demographic and health risk data collected, onsite biometric health screenings, and interest and feedback surveys. Schrader believes that "through the assessment of the wants, as well as the needs of the population(s) you are working with, potential participants in wellness programs become involved in the decision making process" (personal communication). By doing this, you have essentially just engaged them! Schrader has found that by asking employees what they want and examining other data sources to reveal what they need, employees remain engaged in the initiative, programs relevant to employee interests are maintained, and effective health improvement strategies are provided.

Collecting data allows you to gather intelligence on the major health risks of an organization's population so you can target your wellness strategies to generate significant health improvements. Without relevant data collection, and just as important, the evaluation of relevant data, you may fail to offer appropriate programs specific to the needs and wants of your population. Although the collection of relevant data is critical, a potential pitfall is the collection and analysis of too much data. The ACSM states that "we are living in the midst of an information explosion" (Cox, 2003, p. 125) and recommends the development of a targeted strategy based on four or five key pieces of data that provide meaningful information.

Broadening the Understanding of the Actual Determinants of Health

Most wellness initiatives focus on four health behaviors that contribute to 50 percent of annual deaths in the United States: poor nutrition, sedentary lifestyles, tobacco use, and excessive alcohol consumption (Cox, 2003). Although these four high-risk behaviors warrant a great deal of intervention, compelling evidence suggests that a variety of other socioeconomic factors significantly affect people's health, including occupation, work environment (including the quality and quantity of social interaction at work), on-the-job recognition (or lack thereof), income, and education. These factors account for many health disparities within organizations (see chapter 3) and may be root causes of unhealthy behaviors (Cox, 2003).

A better understanding of health determinants may help you take your wellness initiative to the next level by allowing you to tailor it more precisely to the population you serve. This may include incorporating strategies to strengthen social networks, improve work–life balance, create a less stressful work environment, and increase individuals' sense of purpose and value to the organization. Understanding determinants of healthy behaviors means uncovering the *whys* behind, or motivators for, unhealthy behaviors. An assessment of the environment of your organization may assist you with this.

Policy and Environmental Approaches

"It is unreasonable to expect that people will change their behavior easily when so many forces in the social, cultural and physical environment conspire against such change" (Smedley and Syme, 2000, pg. 4). Environmental and policy approaches to wellness and health promotion are based on ecological models of behavior and have the potential to influence behavior change at the population level. Interest in this level has increased over the last decade. Policy and environmental approaches may have greater impact because they influence the overall environment, reach many people, and are less costly and more enduring than clinical, individual, and small-group educational interventions. The U.S. Centers for Disease Control and Prevention (CDC) presents the social-ecological model as a multilevel approach to behavior change (see figure 4.1). In this model, a person's knowledge, skills, attitudes, beliefs, and behaviors are influenced by all levels of society as shown.

Worksite, community, and school environments may be built or adapted to support positive health behaviors. Examples of environmental supports for healthy behaviors include local or on-site farmers markets, walking or biking paths, community gardens, and healthy foods and beverages in vending machines.

Policy Approaches

The smoking ban in public buildings in the United States is one of the most stunning examples of how public health policies can positively affect behavior change (and reduce health risks related to secondhand smoke) in a large number of people. Based on an international study of the cardiovascular effect of public smoking bans, Dr. David Meyers of the University of Kansas School of Medicine stated, "Public smoking bans seem to be tremendously effective in reducing heart attack and, theoretically, might also help to prevent lung cancer and emphysema, diseases that develop much more slowly than heart attacks" (Meyers, Neuberger, He, 2009). Following are a few examples of policies that have been implemented in worksite, community, and school settings to support healthy lifestyle behaviors.

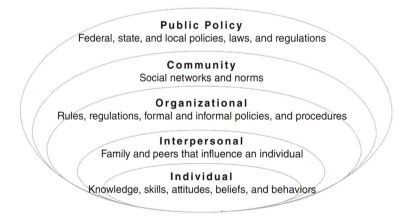

Figure 4.1   Social-ecological model.

From CDC.

Worksites

- Healthy foods and beverages served at meetings, conferences, and events
- Healthy foods and beverages in cafeterias and vending machines
- Time off from work to participate in wellness activities or health screenings
- No-smoking policies

Communities

- Ban of trans fat use in restaurants
- Food stamp acceptance at local farmers markets
- Tax increases on cigarettes and unhealthy foods
- Tax discounts or health insurance co-payment discounts for fitness club memberships

Schools

- Healthy foods and beverages in cafeterias and vending machines
- Reduction or elimination of sugar-sweetened beverages
- Walk-to-school policy on specific days or by students who live within certain distances
- Increase in the frequency or duration of physical education classes

Environmental Approaches

Purchase your access card and pick up a bike to tour or run errands all around the city of Paris. *Vélib'*, a government run bicycle rental program, provides environmental support for increased physical activity by improving bicycle access for city residents as well as tourists. Vélib' aims to combine vélo (bicycle) with liberté (freedom) to transform Parisian transportation while improving health. You can drop off and pick up bicycles at any of the 900 rental stations (soon to be more) strategically placed around the city, regardless of where you originally picked up your bicycle; making the program very convenient. The first half-hour is free, and the second half-hour is one euro, dismissing the perceived barrier of cost and increasing program utilization. Communities around the world are implementing several environmental approaches, such as Vélib', to promote increased physical activity by improving the physical environment. Similar approaches can be implemented in any setting (i.e., worksites, communities, and schools) by making walking trails around buildings and adding bicycle racks, fitness tracks, and playing fields.

Both policy and environmental approaches to wellness and health promotion may result in reaching more people and reaching them more effectively. Some of the following approaches may be easy to implement and low cost, whereas others may require larger investments.

Worksites

- On-site fitness facilities with showers and changing rooms
- Inviting stairwells or other building design features to promote physical activity

- Healthy foods available in on-site cafeterias, snack shops, and vending machines
- Bulletin boards, kiosks, Internet, or other communication mechanisms that provide information on the worksite's wellness initiative, community opportunities for wellness programs, or general health promotion information

Communities

- Crossing guards and bike paths in areas where most pedestrians are children, (e.g., near schools, parks, and playgrounds)
- Sidewalks and pedestrian walkways
- Publicizing local farmers markets to promote the purchase of fresh fruits and vegetables
- Publicizing community-based health education opportunities or groups (e.g., smoking cessation, diabetes education, health fairs or clinics, and physical activity opportunities)

Schools

- Safe walking routes to school
- Playing fields, playgrounds, walking or running tracks or fitness trails
- Farm-to-school programs
- More fruits and vegetables on school breakfast and lunch menus

Benchmarking a Wellness Initiative or Program

If you have an existing wellness initiative, you may be interested in seeing how your program compares against benchmarks or other best-in-class initiatives. The following assessments also reveal best practices in wellness initiatives and health management. These criteria may be applied to most worksite, community, and school settings. The following resources are available to assess or benchmark your wellness initiative:

- The Health Enhancement Research Organization (HERO) provides a scorecard that employers can access, at no charge, to score their wellness initiative and generate a free report. The questions cover program infrastructure, strategy, design, communication, data collection, measurement, and outcomes. The HERO scorecard helps employers learn about best practices in employee health management while helping HERO build a large national database for research and benchmarking purposes. Once you complete the survey, you receive a score that is compared to the aggregated scores in the HERO database (www.the-hero.org/scorecard.htm).

- The National Business Group on Health (NBGH) also offers a wellness impact scorecard for its members. The scorecard is an online tool to help employers evaluate the impact of their wellness or health improvement initiatives on the overall health of their workforce. (See part II of this book for more information.)

- The Wellness Council of America (WELCOA) has benchmarks for successful worksite wellness initiatives. There are four levels of awards an organization can strive to achieve: bronze, silver, gold, and platinum. The criteria for all the awards are based on the progress of the wellness initiative, as compared to WELCOA's seven key benchmarks (www.welcoa.org).

- The U.S. Centers for Disease Control and Prevention (CDC) offers a School Health Index (SHI). "The SHI is a self-assessment and planning tool that schools can use to improve their health and safety policies and programs." The CDC Web site offers a lot of information, including planning guides, training manuals, PowerPoint presentations, and other tools to help improve and assess school-based wellness or health improvement programs (https://apps.nccd.cdc.gov/shi/default.aspx).

- The CDC offers a number of online tools for community assessments. However, many focus on policy and environmental interventions, which, although they merit the attention of seasoned wellness initiatives as indicated earlier, are beyond the scope of this book. To learn more about healthy community assessments and design, visit www.cdc.gov/healthyplaces/. Also, see the School Health Index program in part II.

Summary

Chapter 4 outlines strategies and tools to help you improve and develop an existing wellness initiative. The chapter explains the importance of ensuring that a strong foundation is laid prior to adding on to an existing wellness initiative. Several key questions help you determine the health of your wellness initiative to decide whether your wellness initiative is ready for growth or expansion, or if you must go back to the basics and review the essential components of a wellness initiative detailed in chapters 2 and 3. Strategies to enhance wellness initiatives are presented, and policy and environmental approaches to wellness are introduced. The chapter concludes with benchmarking resources and tools for wellness initiatives.

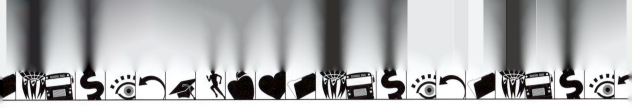

Winning Wellness Programs

The 55 wellness programs presented in part II can assist organizations and individuals in reaching their physical activity and wellness goals as outlined by the National Physical Activity Plan (NPAP) and the Health and Human Services (HHS) Guidelines. These programs may be either implemented as stand-alone programs or used to complement or supplement existing wellness programs or comprehensive wellness initiatives. For example, many worksites, communities, and schools have health insurers or vendors that provide a wide array of online wellness programs. To keep wellness visible in any culture, programs presented in this section may be combined with online programs. This will not only increase interest and engagement in any online wellness programs or services offered, but will also build on any preexisting culture of wellness and improve engagement, health outcomes, and return on investment (ROI).

Any of the programs in this section may be tailored to fit your organizational setting, community, target population, or budget, as well as any seasonal variations, among other factors. You may add your own spices to these recipes for implementing model wellness programs. One size does *not* fit all; therefore, the programs featured in the following chapters vary by setting (worksites, communities, or schools), type (awareness, education, or intervention), topic (nutrition, physical activity, general health and prevention tools), and cost (low, medium, or high). (Chapter 1 details the rationale for implementing wellness programs in worksite, community, and school settings. A combination of awareness, education, and intervention programs may be offered in a comprehensive wellness initiative to attract a wide variety of participants in various stages of change; these types of programs are detailed in chapter 2.)

Chapter 5 features physical activity programs that include one-time awareness and education programs (e.g., Fitness Bee) to longer-term behavior change interventions (e.g., Just Move It). These programs may be applied to a variety of settings as well as fitness levels.

Chapter 6 features nutrition programs, which include awareness, education, and behavior change programs. Free nutrition education programs are also provided that may be implemented in schools, communities, and worksites (e.g., Portion Distortion).

Chapter 7 features general health and preventive programs including education and intervention programs and simple awareness and reminder programs such as Make It Stick. Several fun selections to reduce stress, such as Laugh It Up! and Stress-Less Day, along with evidence-based behavior change interventions, such as Pro-Change, are included.

Each program follows a set structure, which facilitates finding information in all of the programs. Each program begins with a brief introduction followed by a list of program goals. Next, a description tells you how to carry out the program, and an enhancements section (if applicable) offers suggestions for modifying the program to fit your needs. Finally, contact information and resources are provided for many of the programs in case you need more information or want to order program materials.

Each program also displays a series of icons to show you where it is applicable:

 = Community settings. These include city or town recreation departments, community health centers, faith-based organizations, health clubs and fitness centers, hospitals, nonprofit organizations, nursing homes, senior centers, and senior housing.

 = Worksite settings. These include human resources organizations, municipalities, organized labor organizations, private sector worksites, and state and federal government worksites.

 = School settings. These include early childhood centers, schools, universities, and colleges. Programs specific to certain ages or educational levels are identified as such.

 = Awareness programs. These provide reminders, or prompts, along with basic health messages.

 = Education programs. These provide educational materials, lectures, and other resources to enhance participants' knowledge of wellness and health behavior topics. Education programs may be one-time programs or series consisting of multiple sessions.

 = Intervention programs. These include evidence-based health behavior change programs. Program duration is generally 8 to 12 weeks.

 = Low cost (under $100)

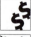 = Medium cost ($100 to $1,000)

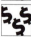 = High cost (greater than $1,000)

(Note that program costs may vary depending on the number of participants and the number and type of enhancements added.)

To help you quickly locate programs that fit your needs, be sure to use the activity finder at the start of the book.

Physical Activity Programs

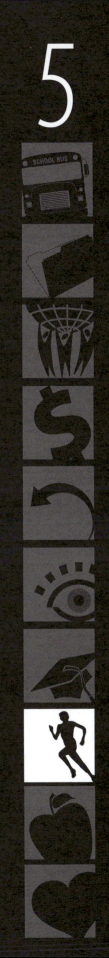

Active Living Every Day

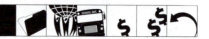

Active Living Every Day is an evidence-based intervention designed to increase daily physical activity. Classes may be taught in person, online, or in combination; and either in groups or with individuals. The barriers to adopting a healthy lifestyle are as varied and complex as the people trying to overcome them. Active Living Partners (ALP) is dedicated to helping people break through those barriers to improve their health and quality of life. Active Living Every Day provides solutions to the problem of getting sedentary adults to become more physically active and make lifestyle changes that will have a positive impact on their lives. There are fees associated with this program; each participant pays $34.95 for a participant package, and the facilitator pays $349 for training.

Goals

- Improve health and quality of life by teaching proven behavior change strategies.
- Teach appropriate lifestyle skills, based on an evidence-based, readiness to change model.
- Assist adults in meeting federal physical activity guidelines.

Description

Active Living Every Day addresses the inherent causes of a sedentary lifestyle and teaches participants the skills they need to identify and overcome their barriers to physical activity, set realistic goals, develop social support, and fit activity into their daily lives. Along the way, they become active by doing activities they enjoy and develop positive feelings about being physically active. Organizations such as fitness centers, worksites, senior residences, community health programs, hospitals, and universities are using Active Living Every Day to empower people to change their health habits. The success the program has had in these varied settings may be traced to the following:

- **Proven effectiveness.** Active Living Every Day was developed in partnership with The Cooper Institute, which has achieved worldwide recognition for its outstanding scientific research, and has been proven effective in clinical trials.
- **Structure and support.** The program structure builds a strong foundation of behavior change and a community of support, providing momentum to extend and entrench each person's wellness habits.
- **Inclusive approach.** Participants build on small successes to create confidence—a method that appeals to even the most sedentary people.
- **Personalized strategies.** The course allows participants to tailor the program based on their readiness to change, lifestyles, and preferences so each person gets the information needed to reach his or her health and fitness goals and make lasting changes.

Equipment and Supplies

- Facilitator package (includes a binder, CD-ROM, online course, and Web site resources)
- Participant package for each person who takes the course (includes a book, online course, and Web site resources)
- Pedometers

Enhancements

- Schedule field trips to local areas of interest, such as parks or activity centers, where participants may be physically active.
- Invite guest speakers to offer additional information based on the program topics.
- Offer physical activity demonstrations outside of class to introduce participants to new activities.

For More Information   Visit www.activeliving.info/, call 1-800-747-4457, or send an e-mail to alpinfo@hkusa.com to learn more about implementing this program.

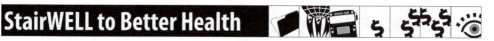
StairWELL to Better Health is a physical activity promotion campaign that raises awareness about the health benefits of taking the stairs versus the elevator. Stair climbing may contribute to weight loss, weight loss maintenance, improved body composition, and building and maintaining healthy bones, muscles, and joints. The number of stairs climbed may be accumulated across the course of the day, making a significant contribution to the recommended 30 minutes of daily physical activity. Evidence suggests that signage may be very effective at improving health behaviors. StairWELL to Better Health may be taken one step further by making physical improvements to stairwells to increase the appeal of taking the stairs, thereby increasing use.

Goals

- Increase physical activity.
- Improve body composition.
- Build and maintain healthy bones, muscles, and joints.

Description   At a children's hospital in Atlanta the stairwells are a preferred way to get to higher floors in the building. The stairwells are very inviting. Piped-in music, beautiful artwork hung on fresh, brightly colored paint, and great lighting all help make the stairwell a pleasant choice over the elevator for staff as well as visitors. Hospital staff observed a higher usage rate since stairwell improvements were completed. It has been reported that many more people use the stairs when prompts and enhancements such as music, photos, and other renovations are made to stairwells.

The U.S. Centers for Disease Control and Prevention's Division of Nutrition, Physical Activity and Obesity (Kerr, Yore, Ham, and Dietz, 2004) conducted a study to determine whether simple improvements in building stairwells, such as adding music and motivational signs, would motivate people to increase their stair use. A four-stage passive intervention was implemented over 42 months and included painting and adding carpeting, framed artwork, motivational signs, and music to stairwells. Infrared beams were used to track the number of stair users. Outcome data suggest that physical improvements, motivational signs, and music do increase stairwell use among building occupants. StairWELL to Better Health may range from a low-cost intervention (e.g., simple motivational signage) to a high-cost intervention (e.g., installing a stairwell music system).

The Web site of the U.S. Centers for Disease Control and Prevention offers many resources to assist in launching a stairwell campaign. They provide information that you may use to "transform your stairs into StairWELLs to Better Health." Topics covered include stairwell appearance, motivational signs, installing music, and tracking stair usage. You may even view before and after photos of renovated stairwells. Visit www.cdc.gov/nccdphp/dnpao/hwi/toolkits/stairwell/index.htm to download, print, and post ready-made signs and additional strategies.

Enhancements

- Design and print your own high-quality posters.
- Laminate your posters for an extra touch, and post on stairwell doors and near elevators.
- Change posters monthly to continue to attract attention.

- Add motivational prompts on each floor (e.g., "Congratulations! You reached level 2!").
- Worksites may launch a 30-day StairWELL to Better Health campaign or competition.
- Distribute promotional materials that outline the benefits of using the stairs.
- Have participants log floors climbed to earn points for reaching certain levels that may be used to receive incentives or prizes (e.g., gift cards).

For More Information   Visit http:///www.cdc.gov/nccdphp/dnpa/hwi/toolkits/ stairwell/index.htm and http://hr.duke.edu/stairwell/ to print a logbook for tracking progress.

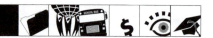

10-10-10 is a wellness program that promotes and provides opportunities for short, accumulated bouts of physical activity in worksite, community, or school settings. The purpose of 10-10-10 is to increase participant awareness of the building body of evidence that suggests that health benefits occur as a result of daily, accumulated, short bouts of exercise. Research findings support the practice of three bouts of 10 minutes of exercise in some populations, and as a strategy to engage people in a physically active lifestyle.

Goals

- Increase physical activity.
- Reduce perceived barrier of lack of time.

Description

Those of us who complain about being time deprived now have no excuse! How many of your clients or employees tell you they would love to exercise, but they do not have the time?

10-10-10 simply makes participants aware of the finding that shorter bouts of exercise have health benefits, and encourages them to engage in some physical activity, even on their busiest days. A study conducted by Schmidt, Biwer, and Kalscheuer (2001) demonstrated that three 10-minute bouts of exercise per day or two 15-minute bouts of exercise per day were just as effective as one 30-minute bout of exercise per day for weight loss and improving fitness levels. The results of this study provide evidence that exercise accumulated in several short bouts has similar effects to one continuous bout with regard to aerobic fitness and weight loss in certain populations. This approach to meeting recommended levels of daily physical activity may assist in reducing barriers to routine physical activity and increase initial engagement. Of course, a daily, continuous, long-term bout of exercise with adherence to various levels of intensity is still considered optimal, but these findings simply suggest that some exercise is better than none. All or nothing is *out*!

Enhancements

- If you are an employer, encourage employees to walk 10 minutes on their morning break, 10 minutes at lunch, and 10 minutes in the afternoon. You may organize group walks (inside and outside the building) to maximize participation.
- If you are a health club owner or personal trainer, use these research findings to get sedentary or inactive people back on track and gradually increase their exercise duration or frequency. Or, you may use it as a "busy day" exercise prescription.
- Schedule a Lunch and Learn to present this evidence, as well as to discuss possible scenarios for achieving short bouts of physical activity throughout the day.
- To promote this program, simply post, e-mail, or mail a flyer that states the health benefits of three 10-minute bouts of exercise over the course of the day, along with helpful suggestions to accomplish this goal. A sample flyer can be found on page 89.

10-10-10

THREE 10-MINUTE BOUTS OF DAILY EXERCISE CAN IMPROVE YOUR HEALTH AND RESULT IN WEIGHT LOSS!

Tips to achieving 10-10-10:

- Take a 10-minute walk on your morning break, at lunch, and before or after dinner.

- Mix and match the following activities to achieve three daily 10-minute exercise intervals:

  Dance to your favorite music

  Take the stairs

  Ride your bike

  Walk your dog

  Jump rope or hula hoop

  Window shop at the mall

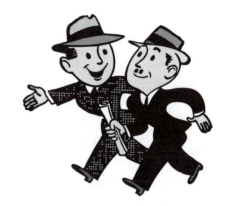

From A. Ludovici-Connolly, 2010, *Winning health promotion strategies* (Champaign, IL: Human Kinetics).

ABC for Fitness

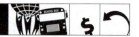

ABC for Fitness, developed by David L. Katz, MD, MPH, and director of the Yale-Griffin Prevention Research Center, is a physical activity program for elementary school students that may be implemented in the classroom throughout the school day.

Goals

- Promote physical activity and health.
- Enhance concentration and the behavioral environment in the classroom.
- Optimize academic performance.

Description   ABC for Fitness (Activity Bursts in the Classroom) is a fun, simple, engaging, no-cost program that uses brief bursts of physical activity during each session of the school day. It is designed to convert the time teachers spend getting restless students to settle down—or distracted students to concentrate—into structured, productive bursts of physical activity spread over the course of the day. Because it fits into small intervals throughout the school day, it is intended to complement rather than replace time spent learning in the classroom. Ideally, the activity bursts will add up to at least 30 minutes of daily physical activity.

ABC for Fitness is offered as approximately five activity bursts of five to six minutes each. However, teachers are encouraged to adapt the length and number of activity bursts to suit their needs and classroom schedules. Each activity burst includes three components: (1) a warm-up using stretches or a low-intensity activity; (2) a core activity, such as jogging in place or dancing, which increases breathing and heart rate; and (3) a cool-down. The program offers a menu of options for warm-ups, core activities, and cool-downs. In addition, it offers guidelines and ideas for four categories of activity bursts: (1) basic activity bursts to provide a break and encourage movement between classes; (2) advanced activity bursts that combine sets of movements into engaging classroom activities; (3) activity bursts of imagination that use the concept of creativity to move in the classroom; and (4) activity bursts for learning and fitness to facilitate hands-on learning in language arts, social studies, music, math, science, and health.

Equipment and Supplies

- ABC for Fitness teacher manual available free of charge at www.davidkatzmd.com/abcforfitness.aspx.
- Optional: Music CDs and CD player
- Optional: Pedometers
- Optional: FitDeck exercise cards
- Some of the learning-related activity bursts require simple equipment such as paper, pencils, markers, index cards, a compass, a wristwatch, masking tape, or a musical instrument.

Enhancements

- Use music to accompany the activity bursts.
- Have students take turn leading the class in activity bursts.
- Incorporate the learning-related activity bursts into your curriculum.

For More Information   Visit www.davidkatzmd.com/abcforfitness.aspx or contact the Yale-Griffin Prevention Research Center at 1-203-732-1265.

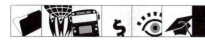

Fitting in Fitness

Fitting in Fitness is a simple e-mail, brochure, or poster awareness campaign that educates participants on simple ways to fit fitness into their daily lives by reducing barriers to exercise, increasing physical activity, and improving the overall health and well-being of those with busy lifestyles.

Goals

- Increase awareness of strategies for fitting in fitness on a regular or daily basis.
- Increase physical activity.
- Reduce barriers to exercise.

Description   The following top 10 strategies for Fitting in Fitness may be e-mailed to employees, provided as a handout, or presented in a 30-minute educational session along with an open discussion of how current participants are fitting fitness into their lives:

1. **Take 10.** Take 10-minute activity breaks three times a day. Research findings support the practice of three accumulated bouts of 10 minutes of exercise as an effective strategy to engage people in a healthy lifestyle. Three accumulated bouts of 10 minutes of exercise equate, in some cases and in some populations, to health benefits similar to those acquired from the recommended 30 minutes of daily physical activity. This approach to meeting recommended levels of daily physical activity may assist in reducing barriers and increase initial engagement. Of course, a daily, continuous, long-term bout of exercise with adherence to various levels of intensity is still considered optimal, but these findings simply suggest that some exercise is better than none. (See 10-10-10 on page 88.)

2. **Walk about.** Energy expenditure accumulates throughout the day the way snowflakes accumulate into blizzards! Take the stairs; park the car farther away; conduct walking meetings; walk the halls at the office and in hotels, airports, and malls. Seek out opportunities to walk about!

3. **Your office gym.** Keep hand weights, a basketball, an exercise band, a jump rope, a yoga mat, a hula hoop, or walking shoes in a basket in your office for daily use.

4. **Recreate yourself.** As life changes, so do your physical activity habits. Revisit recreational activities you may have enjoyed in the past such as ice skating, basketball, softball, hula hooping, or jumping rope, or discover new activities. Recreate yourself through recreation!

5. **Active duty.** Volunteer to help others, perhaps elderly neighbors, by shoveling snow, mowing lawns, or running errands. Volunteer for organizations such as Habitat for Humanity or Meals on Wheels. Contact your church to get the names of community members who may need assistance.

6. **Multitask.** While you are on the phone or watching television, do squats, abdominal exercises, push-ups, or yoga, or dance in the kitchen while you cook. Take a short walk while you brainstorm ideas for a project or work out problems for work.

7. **Recruit troops.** Recruit family, friends, and colleagues. Hire professionals to help you fit in fitness. Ask for help with tasks such as cutting up fruits and vegetables (fun to do with children), pack healthy lunches with your significant other, ask your assistant or colleague to purchase fresh fruit for your office (instead of going out for coffee), or hire a personal trainer to help you develop a targeted, time-efficient routine.

>> *continued*

8. **Schedule health.** Dedicate one morning each week to schedule past-due appointments with health care providers, refill prescriptions, schedule daily fitness activities, and plan meals. Block this time out in your schedule.

9. **Make health a daily priority.** Close the door on your best excuses. We all share common excuses such as no time or energy. Don't allow yourself to let excuses rule your life. Focus on the pros of practicing healthy behaviors. Take charge of your health!

10. **Make fitness fun.** We all find time for what we want to do, for what we find fun. Make sure a fitness program that you enjoy most is on that list. Avoid trying to adhere to obligatory exercise. Rather, make it fun and something you look forward to doing.

Enhancements

- In a group presentation, brainstorm ideas with participants on how they fit fitness into their lives. Share ideas as a group.
- Discuss fitting in healthy eating and other healthy behaviors into a busy lifestyle.
- Provide the list of top 10 strategies for Fitting in Fitness in an e-mail or as a handout for any fitness program, or in any health club or worksite for members.

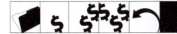

Shape Up the Nation is an online, self-directed physical activity intervention that uses social networks to engage participants. Shape Up the Nation connects people to improve their health collectively. The online platform helps people easily do the following:

- Create and share exercise plans.
- Find someone to work out with.
- Find an intramural sports team to join.
- Find local events and competitions.
- Challenge colleagues to achieve a healthy goal.
- Create a wellness discussion group.
- Recommend a recipe or healthy article.

By harnessing the support of people's trusted social networks—friends, family, and colleagues—Shape Up the Nation helps people eat better, exercise more, stop smoking, or work to achieve almost any health goal they may have. Additionally, the platform enables people and organizations interested in health to connect with each other, providing a single location where people can monitor, manage, and optimize their health. The cost averages $1.00 to $4.00 per employee per month. This can be a high-cost program for the employer if the company covers the program costs.

Goals

- Increase physical activity.
- Promote weight loss.
- Encourage teamwork and peer support.
- Provide a vehicle for people and their physicians, personal trainers or coaches, employers, health insurers, pharmacies, and hospitals to use to communicate.

Description Shape Up the Nation is a wellness program based on medical research that has proven the effectiveness of company health challenges and social networks in improving health. Social incentives rather than financial incentives drive participation.

The platform allows companies to create company-sponsored challenges, groups, and plans. Clients typically launch the program with a 12-week, team-based, company-wide challenge, with employees competing on teams to exercise the most number of minutes, walk the most number of steps, or lose the most weight. Clients often sponsor a series of challenges and events throughout the year, such as a five-a-day fruits and vegetables challenge, a smoking cessation challenge, a stress relief challenge, or a weight management challenge. Shape Up the Nation account managers help clients set up challenges, market them effectively, manage any product fulfillment, evaluate outcomes, and set incentives, if necessary.

The real secret to the success of this program is the everyday interactions of participants. Throughout the year, they create their own challenges and groups and invite each other to activities. The platform makes it easy for participants to create exercise plans (e.g., go to the gym together at 6:00 p.m.) or walking groups. Employees may search for others with similar activity interests or health goals and invite them to an activity or challenge. New employees particularly like the program because it gives them a way to meet people.

>> continued

Participants may also ask one of Shape Up the Nation's experts (e.g., nutritionists and exercise physiologists) any questions about health and wellness. Employees may also share health resources (recipes, books, DVDs, products, and Web sites) with their social networks. They may also learn where their colleagues are working out and band together to get discounts on health products and gym memberships.

The program has been implemented in all types of employee populations and in 26 countries around the world. Many of the tools, such as data reporting, are accessible offline via telephone, SMS text messaging, iPhone, and even paper and pencil. The program has a unique ability to reach employees without computer access as well as tech-savvy smart phone users.

Enhancements   Shape Up the Nation can provide clients with a fully branded and customized version of the program. Clients can opt for customized platforms so they can maintain their internal wellness program's look and feel and integrate it with other wellness offerings, including health risk assessments, telephonic coaching, and incentives.

For More Information   Call 1-877-561-8739, visit http:///www.shapeupthenation. com, or look into local social networking wellness programs in your area.

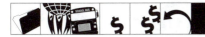

Play Ball is a recreational physical activity program that may include a pickup game of basketball at lunchtime, an organized after-work softball league, a community beach volleyball game, or any other ball game that encourages groups to form to increase physical activity.

Goals

- Increase physical activity by providing recreational opportunities.
- Improve teamwork.
- Create camaraderie and provide social support.

Description

On Tuesdays after work on the lawn of the statehouse, the Department of Environmental Management and the state legislators compete in a friendly game of volleyball. At lunchtime, employees go outdoors to shoot some hoops and discuss a project. Getting outdoors and being active may help clear heads, improve teamwork, and promote a healthy work, community, or school environment. Maintaining a volleyball net for a minimal up-front investment in a community park may help promote physical recreation for adults and children alike. These examples demonstrate how making small additions to a worksite, community, or school environment, such as a basketball net or court, a volleyball net, or simply a lawn designated for badminton, promotes a visual culture of health and wellness by providing access to opportunities for physical activity.

To set up Play Ball, send out an e-mail or post sign-up sheets announcing the program. You may schedule an informational meeting for people who may be interested but are unsure of the level of physical activity and time commitment required. At such a meeting, potential participants can learn about the details of the program and decide whether Play Ball appeals to them. If you just want to offer informal pickup games without sign-ups, simply advertise the days, times, locations, and types of offerings, and encourage participants to come.

Enhancements

- Offices, departments, or communities (e.g., cities or towns) may organize teams to compete.
- Uniforms, new equipment, and charity leagues or competitions may increase the cost of this program.
- Other lawn games may include bocce ball, croquet, a putting green, or Ultimate Frisbee.

Moving Meetings

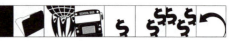

Moving Meetings is a policy program that may be implemented in worksite, community, or school settings to encourage people to move, rather than sit, while they meet. An organization may implement a policy in which two or more people may meet while walking together. Depending on an organization's operating budget and commitment to wellness, treadmill workstations may be purchased to use in conference rooms or offices.

Goals

- Increase physical activity.
- Promote weight loss.
- Maintain weight loss.

Description

As described in chapter 1, employees at Salo are not walking outdoors; they are walking at their treadmill workstations while they work. Employees of Salo have reported significant weight loss by walking at a slow pace of only 1 mile per hour (1.6 km/h) while they work. Walking at this slow pace allows employees to meet and talk on the phone without becoming short of breath.

Don't have funds in the budget for treadmill workstations? Senior leadership can still implement a low-cost policy allowing employees, students, or community groups to conduct moving meetings. A Moving Meetings policy may stipulate that permission must be granted by a supervisor, that only one moving meeting can occur per day, or that moving meetings are restricted to 30 minutes per meeting. By instituting a formal policy, an organization may encourage walking, or moving, meetings instead of meeting in a traditional conference room. Schools may put this program in place as well; for example, teachers can take students on a walk to a local park to review test results or have other lessons or meetings. Staff of community organizations, senior centers, hospitals, nonprofit organizations, and municipalities may all move while meeting.

Enhancements

- Encourage employees to keep an exercise journal to document all walking meetings (set a weekly or hourly walking meeting goal).
- Provide incentives to reach goals.
- Employers can purchase treadmill workstations, deduct the cost from employees' paychecks, or provide them as incentives or bonuses.
- Employers may match employees' contributions to the cost of treadmill workstations or cover the cost of employee participation in a series of wellness initiatives.

For More Information

Visit these Web sites:

- www.salollc.com/
- www.mayoclinic.com/health/office-exercise/SM00115
- www.usatoday.com/tech/news/2005-06-07-office-fit_x.htm?csp=34

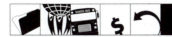

A low cost, six-week physical activity challenge, Just Move It is a self-directed wellness program that can be tailored to individual physical activity preferences. Weekly group meetings are organized to provide hands-on learning related to physical fitness and social support through group discussions, as well as to ensure individual accountability through the submission of physical activity logs with low-cost incentives offered.

Goals

- Increase physical activity.
- Promote weight loss.
- Maintain weight loss.
- Provide opportunities for social support.

Description   Just Move It is a self-directed, six-week physical activity challenge that can be implemented in a variety of settings. A kickoff event both promotes the program and recruits participants. Once enrolled, participants engage in whatever type of physical activity they enjoy, such as walking, biking, or working out in a gym. Group meetings are organized once a week for physical activity workshops, social support, and accountability. Throughout the week, participants exercise independently, in groups, or with an exercise partner, and track their progress by completing a physical activity log (see page 99 for a sample activity log). To promote accountability, participants hand in their physical activity logs as well as reports on their progress at six consecutive weekly meetings.

Here is a weekly schedule to follow:

Week 1: Provide challenge sign-up, an introduction, and a program overview, and obtain signed participant release forms.

Week 2: Interactively introduce ways to increase physical activity, distribute a physical activity tip sheet (see page 98 for a sample tip sheet), and ask participants to add their ideas to this tip sheet, to be updated weekly.

Week 3, 4, and 5: Presentation by guest instructor, group meeting or discussion, physical activity workshop.

Week 6: Final results: Awards presented by administrative host.

At the end of each weekly session, participants complete evaluation forms to both track attendance and evaluate program satisfaction and effectiveness. (See chapter 2 for more information on program evaluation.)

Equipment and Supplies

- Space to accommodate a kickoff event
- Room set up with classroom-style chairs for enrollment session and group meetings
- Additional room set up for physical activity workshops
- Printed and posted promotional materials

>> continued

- Incentives for program completion
- Printed physical activity logs
- Guest instructors for six-week sessions. Guest instructors may include local certified exercise trainers, personal trainers, representatives of local health clubs, representatives of state or local health departments, representatives of state or local parks and recreation departments, and representatives of nonprofit organizations. You may often recruit volunteer guest instructors who benefit from the opportunity to promote their services. Following are five tips on recruiting volunteer guest instructors:
    - Call your local health club, YMCA, hospital, or university.
    - Ask health insurers, local doctors, nurses, or specialists.
    - Invite nonprofit organizations to come in to discuss health concerns specific to your population (e.g., American Diabetes Association or American Heart Association).
    - Find out if anyone working in the organization is a certified exercise instructor.
    - Look into local outdoor clubs to organize hiking, biking, kayaking, and other outdoor activities.
- Participant sign-up sheet and process (e.g., call or e-mail the program facilitator)
- Kickoff event to introduce participants to the program, have them complete necessary paperwork including release forms, and distribute program materials

Enhancements Provide incentives for participation or submission of logs.

Sample Physical Activity Tip Sheet

- Take the stairs.
- Park your car farther away from your destination.
- Walk your dog or offer to walk your neighbor's dog.
- Take a family walk after dinner.
- Go hiking this weekend.
- Ride your bike to work.
- Go for a walk during lunch.
- Wear a pedometer.
- Exercise with a friend.
- Take extra trips around the office.
- Take the long way when walking home.
- Make a daily commitment to move more.

From A. Ludovici-Connolly, 2010, *Winning health promotion strategies* (Champaign, IL: Human Kinetics).

My Physical Activity Tracker

For the week of _____

My goal for this week is:	Cardio (aerobic) exercise for 30 minutes most days of the week	Strength training at least two days a week
Monday Notes to myself:	**Today's goal:** My activities:	**Today's goal:** My activities:
Tuesday Notes to myself:	**Today's goal:** My activities:	**Today's goal:** My activities:
Wednesday Notes to myself:	**Today's goal:** My activities:	**Today's goal:** My activities:
Thursday Notes to myself:	**Today's goal:** My activities:	**Today's goal:** My activities:
Friday Notes to myself:	**Today's goal:** My activities:	**Today's goal:** My activities:
Saturday Notes to myself:	**Today's goal:** My activities:	**Today's goal:** My activities:
Sunday Notes to myself:	**Today's goal:** My activities:	**Today's goal:** My activities:

- **Cardio or aerobic exercise:** Moderate physical activity—You feel your heart beat faster and you breathe faster too. Vigorous physical activity—You have a large increase in breathing and heart rate. Conversation is difficult or broken.
- **Strength training:** Sometimes called resistance exercise; you work your muscles against resistance using weights or gravity (for example, push-ups). Try six to eight strength-training exercises of 8 to 12 repetitions of each exercise.

To track your physical activity online, visit www.presidentschallenge.org.

From A. Ludovici-Connolly, 2010, *Winning health promotion strategies* (Champaign, IL: Human Kinetics). Activity tracker reprinted from www.health.gov/dietaryguidelines/dga2005/healthieryou/html/phys_activity_tracker.html

SparkPeople

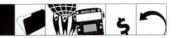

SparkPeople is one of the fastest growing health Web sites in the world, with a mission to spark millions of people to reach their goals and make the world a healthier place—one person at a time. SparkPeople.com is the program's flagship site built for people looking for a diet or healthy living program and community. The purpose of SparkPeople is to increase physical activity, improve nutrition, and promote weight loss. An added benefit is the social networking opportunities for members. This program is free for individuals, but there is a low cost for organizations.

Goals

- Increase physical activity.
- Promote weight loss.
- Maintain weight loss.
- Provide opportunities for social support.

Description

Quilters from across the country gather, discuss their common passion for quilting, and work together as a team to reduce their weight. These quilters are gathering virtually on the SparkPeople Web site. They discuss their common interest in quilting, but also support each other with their weight-loss goals.

Over 5 million people have joined SparkPeople. Founder and CEO, Chris Downey, combines strategies to improve both body and mind in the program. Resources for a healthier body include a wealth of timely information on nutrition and exercise. SparkPeople employs goal setting, motivational techniques, and other strategies to empower people to change their mind-set to achieve their personal weight-loss goals. "SparkPeople is my prescription of choice for patients who need to lose weight," a physician once informed Chris Downey after treating several patients who were achieving positive results through the program.

Enhancements

- Organizations may hold a program launch meeting to explain the program, provide a Web site demonstration, and help people organize teams.
- Various departments, locations, or divisions within an organization may form teams and compete against each other.
- For a small fee, organizations can obtain comprehensive reports and data on team results.

For More Information

Visit http:///www.sparkpeople.com/.

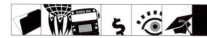

Join the Club is a one-hour awareness and education program designed to provide fitness education as well as increase knowledge of the benefits of joining a health club. Join the Club is a workshop that helps reduce barriers to joining a health club, such as feeling intimidated by current members (even people already planning to join a club may experience this).

Goals

- Increase knowledge of fitness.
- Increase awareness of the benefits of joining a health club.

Description

When I owned a health club, I scheduled an open house every year, typically in January. The public was invited to come to the club for free Join the Club educational lectures provided by local physicians, staff, and members. The staff provided a tour of the facility and lectures on the benefits of strength training, aerobic exercise, and general fitness. Local physicians spoke on the importance of exercise and the positive health benefits associated with regular physical activity. Five to ten current members provided testimonials on their stunning results, both weight-loss and health outcomes. Exercise demonstrations were given and refreshments were served, providing a networking opportunity for dialogue and discussion. Join the Club for free was extremely successful at getting people who may not have felt comfortable walking into a health club on their own to visit or join.

Join the Club may also be implemented in worksite, community, or school settings. Bring in a few representatives from local health clubs to provide a slideshow and talk about their facilities, and to give out free daily or weekly passes. This allows potential members to ask questions and learn about the amenities of the club, which may result in their feeling more comfortable about what they would be walking into.

Enhancements

- Contact local health clubs in your area and request a guest speaker.
- Send out an e-mail or post program information.
- Clubs may offer discounts to anyone who attends the event.
- Offer a complimentary trial workout that day as a taste test. This may be done if the program is offered at the health club. If sufficient room is available, stretching and other exercises may also be offered.
- Join the Club may run all day on a Saturday, or during evenings for several weeks.

For More Information

Contact the International Health, Racquet and Sportsclub Association (IHRSA) at http://cms.ihrsa.org/ to find quality health clubs in your area.

Fitness Bee

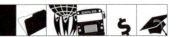

Fitness Bee is an educational program that is designed to increase knowledge of fitness and exercise facts. Fitness Bee may be offered in a variety of settings including worksites, communities, and schools. This one-hour program developed by the director of the Rhode Island State Office of Rehabilitation Services, Steven Brunero, and his wellness team may be offered as a Lunch and Learn wellness activity.

Goals

- Increase knowledge of fitness.
- Increase knowledge of exercise.

Description   Fitness Bee is based on the game show *Truth or Dare* and engages participants by asking them to provide answers to questions on fitness and exercise. Prizes are awarded for correct responses. Questions for Fitness Bee may be developed by the wellness director or the wellness champions. The questions may be developed as a team effort. The person, or team, that answers the most questions correctly wins the Fitness Bee. Following are some sample questions and answers:

Sample Questions and Answers   The following questions and answers are from the American Council on Exercise:

Question 1: If someone sweats during an aerobic workout, is he or she out of shape?

Answer: No. The reason for sweating is that body core temperature becomes elevated by the increase in metabolic heat production during exercise.

Question 2: Does regular participation in aerobic exercise lower an individual's risk of developing cancer?

Answer: Research suggests that exercise often modifies some of the risk factors associated with certain kinds of cancer. Obesity, for example, has been linked to cancer of the breast and the female reproductive system.

Question 3: What is HbA1c, and what does it measure?

Answer: The HbA1c (glycosylated hemoglobin) test measures the amount of glucose that attaches to red blood cells. The higher your blood glucose level, the more sugar your blood cells will accumulate over time. Because the typical life span of red blood cells is 90 to 120 days, the HbA1c test reflects your average blood glucose level over that time period. As a result, it measures how well your blood sugar has been controlled over a period of a few months.

Question 4: What are the benefits of varying your workout routine?

Answer: Varying your workout routine (1) prevents boredom associated with doing the same things workout after workout and (2) avoids or delays reaching a plateau in workout performance and, subsequently, training results. Research also suggests that adding variety to an exercise program may improve adherence.

Question 5: How important are the warm-up and cool-down portions of a workout?

Answer: Warm-up and cool-down activities should be an essential part of all exercise programs. Warm-up activities prepare the body for the conditioning phase of the exercise session. The cool-down phase assures that venous (blood) return to the heart is maintained in the face of significant amounts of blood going to the previously working muscles.

Enhancements

- Fitness Bee may be tailored to include a Nutrition Bee or a General Health Bee.
- Schedule Fitness Bee at lunchtime in the worksite, during class time in school, or in the evening at a community center.
- Advertise Fitness Bee and offer small prizes or incentives for teams or individuals who win.
- Fitness Bee can be offered in a variety of different ways. Offer Fitness Bee for a designated period of time such as six to eight consecutive weeks, or offer it as a one-time event.
- Include Fitness Bee as part of a health fair or other wellness event or program.
- If Fitness Bee is offered as part of a Lunch and Learn wellness program, a healthy lunch may be served.

For More Information   Visit www.cdc.gov/ for potential question content organized by health topics.

Let's Dance

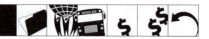

Let's Dance is an eight-week physical activity intervention or dance program that engages large groups of people in worksite, community, or school settings. While increasing physical activity and learning a variety of dances, participants also develop social relationships at these events.

Goals

- Increase physical activity.
- Provide opportunities for social support.

Description   The city of Nashville, Tennessee, offers large groups of people the opportunity to improve physical activity by offering weekly dance events. In addition to increasing weekly physical activity and learning a variety of dances, participants develop social relationships through Let's Dance. Worksites, communities, and schools may offer this consecutive, eight-week dance program. Each week a different local band may volunteer to provide music, or a local DJ or stereo may be substituted. Dance themes and music and dance instruction may change weekly, keeping the program interesting. These events, which may run for up to three hours weekly, provide community members with an excellent opportunity to gather, socialize, and exercise!

To implement this program, you'll need to ensure adequate space, including an indoor location in the event of rain, to accommodate bands and dancing. Find local bands or disc jockeys who will volunteer to provide dance music in exchange for promotion and exposure. If necessary, you can substitute a stereo system. Dance instructors from local dance studios may also be willing to volunteer.

Enhancements   Additional program enhancements will require more advanced planning and coordination but may include the following:

- Provide other health awareness opportunities each week. For example, local hospitals or health insurers may provide preventive health screenings or health information.
- Offer local healthy foods for sale by local restaurants or caterers.
- Conduct a brief post survey of participants to track attendance and evaluate program satisfaction (see the sample survey in chapter 2).
- Schools may offer weekly local bands with no dance instruction to provide children with freestyle dance opportunities.
- Offer cultural dance themes. Despina Metakos, wellness champion from the Department of Transportation in Rhode Island and Jean Kapetanios, from UnitedHealthcare, volunteered their time to lead a Greek dance class, OPA!, for state employees after work hours. Employees learned a different Greek dance each week for six weeks.
- Local bands or disc jockeys may sell their CDs.
- Dance instructors may provide instruction sheets so participants can practice at home throughout the week.

Nutrition Programs

6

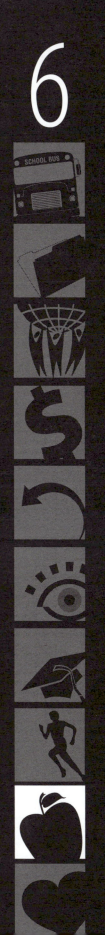

Nutrition Detectives

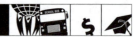

Nutrition Detectives is a 90-minute educational program that teaches children five clues to help them make healthy food choices and detect marketing deceptions by using food labels and ingredient lists. It includes a PowerPoint slideshow, a food demonstration, and a hands-on activity in which children examine food products. The program is also available on DVD. This program is most appropriate for elementary school children.

Goals

- Teach children to make healthy food choices.
- Teach children how to detect marketing deceptions.

Description

Nutrition Detectives is an exciting nutrition education program for elementary school children. It provides a novel, creative, engaging, and efficient way to impart crucial information in minimal time. The program shows children how to read food labels and detect marketing deceptions, while learning to identify and choose healthy foods. It has been taught in schools throughout the United States.

Nutrition Detectives was developed by David Katz, MD, MPH, director of the Yale-Griffin Prevention Research Center, and his wife, Catherine Katz, PhD. The program uses a slideshow with colorful cartoons and images to convey the concept of healthy eating and the challenges of healthy eating in our modern environment. The slideshow shows children how food packages may be deceptive and how nutrition facts labels may be used to make better choices. It provides five clues to make healthy food choices by using food labels and ingredient lists on packaged foods. Children are taught to look for key ingredients such as partially hydrogenated oils, high-fructose corn syrup, and fiber.

The slideshow is followed by a demonstration in which the ingredients of a highly processed food are poured onto a plate. After learning the clues, the children are assigned to teams that take part in a hands-on "spying on food labels" game. Each team searches through a bag of groceries filled with packaged foods. Each bag contains both "clued-in" (healthy) and "clueless" (less healthy) food products, and the children work together to decide which foods fit into each category.

Equipment and Supplies

- A laptop computer, LCD projector, and screen
- Microsoft PowerPoint software
- Nutrition Detectives PowerPoint slideshow and teacher manual
- Grocery bags
- Markers to label each bag
- Groceries as specified in the Play With Our Food section of the manual
- Optional: A stop-watch to initiate and time the hands-on activity

Enhancements

- The program may be taught in one, two, or three sessions depending on the needs of the program provider.
- Give students the opportunity to sample the healthy food products after the activity.
- Photocopy a single-page list of the five clues for each child (see the teacher manual).
- Photocopy a set of five pages describing each clue (see the teacher manual).
- Purchase optional props such as detective hats and sunglasses from inexpensive supply houses or Internet sites such as Rhode Island Novelty (http://rinovelty.com) or Oriental Trading Company (www.orientaltrading.com).
- Offer the program to parents or guardians of the children.

For More Information Preview the materials at www.davidkatzmd.com/nutritiondetectives.aspx and download the teacher manual and slideshow. For additional information, contact the Yale-Griffin Prevention Research Center at 203-732-1265.

Portion Distortion

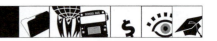

Portion Distortion is a portion-control awareness and education program developed by the National Heart, Lung and Blood Institute. The program teaches skills for proper portion control, identified in research as a key strategy for weight control. Portion Distortion may be augmented by the addition of visual aids and nutrition education.

Goals

- Increase awareness of the importance of portion sizes.
- Increase knowledge of and skills for choosing proper portion sizes in food preparation and consumption.

Description

Portion Distortion is a PowerPoint slide presentation that may be coupled with an educational display set up on a single 8-foot (2.4 m) table in a high-traffic, strategic location such as outside a cafeteria or in a main lobby. The program may be offered as a stand-alone stop-by event, or coupled with a larger event such as a health fair, biometric screening, or farmers market. (The PowerPoint slide presentation could also be shown at a meeting, during lunch, or as part of another event.) The PowerPoint presentation, developed by the National Heart, Lung and Blood Institute's Obesity Education Initiative, is projected from a laptop onto a screen, or may be viewed from the laptop itself. The presentation can be set up to run continuously so visitors can come by and view it at their leisure. Along with the presentation, a table is set up with educational materials, visuals, and samples of proper portion sizes. Here are some labeled visual aids you may use to demonstrate proper portion sizes:

One tennis ball = 1 cup cooked pasta or rice

Four dice = 1.5 oz hard cheese

One deck of cards = 3 oz steak, chicken, or pork

One checkbook = 3 oz fish fillet

One shot glass = 2 Tbsp salad dressing

One die = 1 tsp butter or margarine

One 2-oz. Dixie cup = 1 oz of nuts

One baseball = 1 cup of raw leafy vegetables

One lightbulb = 1/2 cup of vegetables

One cell phone = 1/2 cup fruit

One makeup compact = 1 cookie

One hockey puck = 1/2 a medium bagel

Supplies

- Laptop and LCD projector
- Eight-foot (2.4 m) table

Enhancements

- Provide nutritional handouts, weight-loss information, and resources.
- Gather food replicas as described.

For More Information

Visit http://hp2010.nhlbihin.net/portion/ to download the free slide sets. To order a Food Replicas Starter Kit, visit http:///www.enasco.com/product/WA09755E.

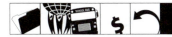

Farmers markets may be offered in a wide variety of settings. Market size may vary from one farm stand to several, depending on the setting, available space, and potential number of consumers. Farmers markets have proven to significantly reduce reported barriers to fruit and vegetable consumption by improving physical access to high-quality, fresh produce at affordable prices (Cyzman, Wierenga, and Sielawa, 2009).

Goals

- Improve access to fresh fruits and vegetables.
- Increase fruit and vegetable consumption.

Description

On a warm summer afternoon at 30 Rockefeller Center in New York City, you may find dozens of farmers displaying their produce under a sea of white top tents. Local farmers proudly display colorful fresh fruits and vegetables, fragrant freshly cut flowers, and homemade jellies and jams, while shoppers carefully make their selections with smiles on their faces. The city coordinates this event for 10 weeks throughout the summer for its residents and workers. This market is a huge success! This is just one example of how farmers markets have changed the health and wellness landscape in worksite, community, and school settings. From one farm stand outside a diner in New Hampshire on a summer Saturday afternoon, to the multiple farmers who come out midweek in New York City, farmers markets are cropping up in the most likely and unlikely places. They are becoming increasingly recognized as an effective nutrition intervention to increase fruit and vegetable consumption.

Any worksite, community, or school may offer a farmers market, or stand, of any size. You may contact a single local farmer and have one small stand on site one day per week, or check with your state department of agriculture or environmental management about offering a larger-scale market. You may feature in-season fruits, vegetables, and flowers. To have a larger farmers market, you may have to partner with other local organizations. For example, a worksite may be in the vicinity of other worksites or businesses that may be interested in collectively sponsoring a farmers market. A health club or community center may have enough traffic to justify a Saturday farmers market, particularly if it is centrally located among other community-based organizations that may participate. A farmers market may also generate new business or increase membership in a health club or community center by attracting people who may otherwise not have been in the area.

Enhancements

- Partner with local culinary schools or chefs to offer cooking demonstrations at the markets.
- Offer food or recipe samples featuring in-season fruits or vegetables. For example, if blueberries are in season, offer samples of blueberry yogurt and granola parfaits.
- Engage the audience in brief physical activity demonstrations at the markets.

For More Information

- Contact your state department of agriculture or environmental management.
- Contact local farmers near your worksite, community, or school to see if they would be willing to set up an on-site market one day per week.

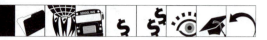

Lunch and Learn is a low-cost (approximately $10 per person) nutrition awareness and education program that engages participants and senior leaders to learn about healthy food choices while enjoying a healthy lunch together.

Goals

- Increase awareness and knowledge about nutrition and healthy food choices.
- Provide an opportunity for participants to eat a nutritious, low-calorie lunch.
- Demonstrate senior-level support of healthy food choices for employees or students.

Description   Lunch and Learn is a nutrition program that raises awareness and provides education on healthy eating in a group setting. It may be incorporated into a variety of settings including worksites; community-based organizations such as community centers, hospitals, and health clubs; and schools. Lunch and Learn is a one-hour nutrition program that may be held during lunch hour once a week for 8 to 12 weeks, or any frequency appropriate for an organization.

This program may involve more advanced planning, so here are some tips to keep in mind:

- Check the calendars of senior leadership, get an advanced commitment from them to attend, and choose date(s) that avoid busy times of the year such as holiday seasons. You may invite special guests, community leaders, or public officials to participate in the program.
- The location for the program should be a conference room, lobby, or other location where participants may sit as well as stand and socialize.
- Decide on a menu and budget. Obtain estimates from local caterers or restaurants that may provide discounts on lunch for free advertising or service promotion. Check with the members of your organization to see whether anyone has connections with a local caterer or restaurant that may be willing to provide healthy lunches at a discount.
- Hire a caterer or offer a healthy potluck lunch by asking each employee, student, or community member to bring in a healthy lunch dish. Advanced sign-ups for certain items will allow for better meal planning.
- Purchase tablecloths, cutlery, plates, napkins, and other necessary items.
- Ask each member to also bring in a less healthy lunch option to display on a side table with a note card describing its nutritional content to educate people of these less healthy alternatives.
- Ensure that space is reserved, and that tables and chairs are available.
- Advertise the program.
- Participants may be charged for the program (e.g., $10 each) or may contribute a healthy item to the program in the form of a potluck. Alternatively, an organization may sponsor the entire program. Have a wellness champion serve as the key contact person for organizing the event and collecting fees.
- Ask the caterer, restaurant, or your wellness team to provide note cards displaying the nutritional content of each item served as well as the nutritional content

of higher-calorie alternatives, if possible (e.g., mustard versus mayonnaise or different salad dressings).

- Stage the program with balloons, decorations, music, or other appealing items; or feature a theme.

Enhancements

- You may enhance the program by offering it weekly for 12 weeks and changing the menu frequently to provide more education about healthy lunch alternatives.
- Hold the program on weekends at health clubs, community centers, or other locations.
- Healthy Holiday Meal, Healthy Fast Food, or Healthy Dinner programs may also be offered.

Drink Up: A Hydration Challenge

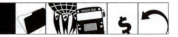

Drink Up is a hydration challenge designed to increase daily water intake. Drink Up may be offered at health clubs, worksites, schools, senior centers, and many other settings. There are many well-documented health benefits of daily adequate water intake. Despite these benefits, many Americans still do not meet the recommendation of six to eight 8-ounce (237 ml) glasses of water per day.

Goals

- Raise awareness of current and recommended water intake.
- Increase water intake to meet daily recommendation.

Description
Purchase promotional water bottles imprinted with your wellness brand name or logo. (Contact promotional vendors and obtain quotes on what these might cost.) The water bottles not only serve as an incentive for the challenge, but assist with the promotion and marketing of your wellness initiative as members carry their bottles with them to various places throughout the day. Distribute water bottles to members who sign a Drink Up challenge agreement to meet the daily recommended water intake of six to eight 8-ounce glasses per day for one week to one month. (A sample challenge agreement is provided on page 113.) Be sure to schedule a kickoff day and sign-ups. Send participants e-mail reminders and motivational tips.

Enhancements

- Supplement the program with nutritional lectures. Explain the benefits of adequate water intake and the effects of various beverages (e.g., water, coffee, sugar-sweetened beverages, energy drinks) on hydration status and body functioning.

- Offer a program enhancement such as a six-week challenge. Provide an added incentive to anyone who completes the enhanced challenge.

- Provide spring water service on site, in a highly visible area, to support program adherence and eliminate any barriers to water access. Promote the challenge at the water cooler.

- Institute an organizational policy to offer water and other beverages low in added sugars (e.g., 100 percent fruit juices, low-fat or non-fat milk, and regular and decaffeinated coffee or tea) in vending machines. Consider a policy to eliminate soda and other sugar-sweetened beverages from vending machines.

Drink Up Challenge Agreement

I [INSERT NAME] agree to participate in the Drink Up Hydration Challenge and agree to meet the daily recommended water intake of six to eight 8-ounce glasses of water for one month beginning _____ [INSERT DATE] and ending _____ [INSERT DATE].

Signature: _____ Date: _____

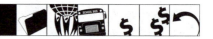

An Apple a Day is a nutrition intervention program. Participants who eat an apple each day at work, school, or a community-based organization such as a community center or health club for 21 consecutive days receive an incentive such as a raffle ticket.

Goals

- Increase apple (fruit) consumption.
- Educate participants on the benefits of eating apples (fruit).

Description   A bushel of shiny, delicious apples is prominently displayed on a table next to the front desk, and employees are encouraged to take one each day for the month of September. (Contact local orchards to obtain discounted rates on apples, or encourage participants to bring their own apple in each day.) Employees get Apple a Day cards punched each day they eat an apple. (See the bottom of this page for a punch card you can use.) At the end of the 21 days, anyone who hands in a completed punch card is entered into a raffle. Apple recipes are also provided each week to help employees continue eating apples by providing a variety of options for preparing or cooking with apples. This type of intervention is effective because it reinforces education (i.e., learning about the benefits of apple consumption) with the desired behavior change (i.e., increased apple consumption).

Enhancements

- Contact local registered dietitians or nutritionists in private practice or at your state or local health departments or universities, or contact your local culinary college or any college in your area that offers a culinary arts program, for handouts on the benefits of eating apples and other fruits and vegetables, recipes, or on-site cooking demonstrations.
- Recipe boards may be hung in various locations for participants to share apple recipes.
- This program may be just a one-day awareness event at which apples, recipes, and handouts on their health benefits are distributed.

For More Information   Visit www.fruitsandveggiesmatter.gov/ to read about the benefits of eating apples (fruit) and for creative recipes.

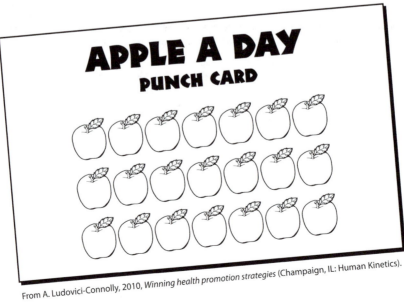

From A. Ludovici-Connolly, 2010, *Winning health promotion strategies* (Champaign, IL: Human Kinetics).

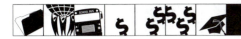

The Community Cookbook program may be implemented in worksite, community, and school settings. Healthy recipes, contributed by participants, are compiled, posted, and printed in a bound Community Cookbook for distribution.

Goals

- Improve nutrition.
- Increase the number of meals prepared at home.
- Help create a culture of community wellness.

Description   Community Cookbook may be implemented in a variety of settings. Employees, members of community-based organizations, or students may be asked to submit their favorite healthy recipe. Request for submissions may be in the form of an e-mail, mailing, newsletter, or bulletin board. One person may serve as the contact person who collects and reviews submissions for posting and printing. You may ask a member of your wellness team or a registered dietitian or nutritionist (if you have access to one) to review recipe submissions for nutritional content.

A bulletin board promoting Community Cookbook may be placed at the entrance of a building. Blank index cards and pushpins are placed on a small table next to the board. Participants are encouraged to either take an index card and return it with their favorite healthy recipe and their name written on it, or write their recipe on the card at that time. Recipes are then posted on the board. Leaders may launch this program by posting at least one of their favorite healthy recipes from the very start, demonstrating senior leader support. Don't post a bare Community Cookbook or bulletin board. People will be more apt to become engaged in the process by seeing current postings. Recipe compilation may also be done online with adequate program promotion. The advantage of online submissions is the ease in cutting and pasting content for print. Consider recruiting volunteers or students (e.g., in nutrition, dietetics, health education, or nursing programs) to assist.

Recipes may be collected over a period of three or four weeks. It may take an additional four weeks to evaluate and format acceptable submissions for the posting of the recipes and the printing of the Community Cookbook.

The fee for the cookbook may vary. Cookbooks may be provided as an incentive at no cost to contributors, or at no cost to employees as part of a healthy eating initiative. A nominal fee may be charged to cover the cost of printing. The printing may be done in house and spiral bound, if resources are available, or sent to a local printer. The cost of each cookbook may run from $5 to $25 depending on the size of the cookbook, the quality of the printing, the cover selection, colors, and other factors.

Enhancements

- Provide an incentive to each person contributing a recipe.
- Arrange for a registered dietitian or nutritionist to analyze the nutritional content of the recipes.
- Ask a well-respected health care professional from the community to write a preface for the Community Cookbook that acknowledges community contributions and emphasizes the importance of a healthy diet and home-cooked meals.
- Ask a community leader (e.g., worksite CEO, city or town mayor, school principal, or superintendent) to write a foreword for the Community Cookbook.
- Offer a community fund-raising event at which people can sample the recipes and purchase the cookbook.

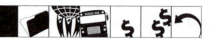

Many workers consume a significant portion of their food intake away from home. Healthy Meetings is a policy program designed to increase the consumption of healthy foods and beverages at breaks or at meals at meetings, conferences, and other work-related events. This program simply requires senior leaders to write and implement a policy that healthy foods and beverages be served at all meetings and events. A link to a sample of a Healthy Meeting policy is provided later.

Goals

- Make healthy food more readily available at gatherings.
- Increase the consumption of healthy foods and beverages during the workday, during the school day, or at public, community-based events.

Description

To address the national obesity epidemic, a state organization gathered more than 150 representatives from community-based organizations at a statewide health conference to develop a comprehensive plan to prevent and reduce obesity and related chronic diseases. Attendees arrived early at the hotel hosting the conference to socialize with their colleagues and have a buffet breakfast prior to the welcoming of attendees and the keynote address. Buffet selections included coffee, tea, juice, scrambled eggs, French toast, muffins, plain and chocolate chip pancakes, bacon, and sausage. There was not a fresh fruit or vegetable in sight. This was a contradictory message to give attendees about the very purpose of the meeting.

Kathleen Cullinen, PhD, RD, LDN, former director of the Rhode Island Obesity Prevention and Control Program, stated, "As health professionals, it is critical to practice what we preach by instituting health policies and creating healthy environments to support and enhance individual efforts to eat a healthy diet and lead a healthy lifestyle." Making healthy food available at work-related events is one way to encourage employees to eat a healthy diet. The U.S. Centers for Disease Control and Prevention (CDC) has established guidelines for healthier eating at work-related events. These guidelines may be used for selecting healthy foods and beverages for breaks or meals at meetings, conferences, and other work-related events. When planning menus, consider providing options that accommodate various dietary preferences and needs.

- Offer a variety of grains—especially whole grains—and fruits and vegetables. Examples include whole-grain breads, pasta, and cereals; fresh fruit and salads; and fresh and cooked vegetables.
- Provide fat-free, low-fat, or low-calorie foods and beverages. Ideas include grilled or roasted entrees; fat-free or low-fat dressings or toppings such as salsa, low-fat yogurt dressing, and sweet mustard; low-fat or low-calorie desserts such as angel food cake; low-fat or skim milk, low-fat yogurt or cheese; and lean meats, poultry or fish, beans, peas, and lentils.
- Offer foods and beverages low in added sugars. You may serve unsweetened cereals, fruit spreads, water, 100 percent fruit juices, diet drinks, low-fat or non-fat milk, and regular and decaffeinated coffee or tea.
- Serve foods that are low in sodium. These include food items such as unsalted pretzels and popcorn, entrees made with herbs and spices instead of salt, and fresh foods instead of processed foods that tend to be high in sodium.

- Include smaller portions. Examples include mini-muffins or mini-bagels, 1-inch (2.5 cm) low-fat cheese squares, and small beverages.
- Offer only beverages at midmorning and midafternoon breaks.

The cost for this program varies from low (e.g., encouraging meeting participants to bring healthy food to share from home) to high (e.g., having the organization cover the entire cost of healthy foods and beverages served at all meetings and conferences). For a sample Healthy Meetings policy from North Carolina's Eat Smart Program, visit www.co.nash.nc.us/LinkClick.aspx?fileticket=8SybvOW0PRQ%3D&tabid=1011. This template may be tailored for any organization, agency, or community group where foods or beverages are served.

Enhancements

- Post nutrition and calorie information at point-of-purchase or serving areas.
- Offer healthy foods and beverages in cafeterias.
- Offer healthy foods and beverages in vending machines.

For More Information   For more information on Healthy Meeting policies, please refer to the following resources:

- U.S. Department of Health and Human Services and U.S. Department of Agriculture. 2005, January. *Dietary Guidelines for Americans, 2005*. 6th ed., Washington, DC: U.S. Government Printing Office. Available at www.health.gov/dietaryguidelines.

- American Public Health Association Policy Statement 9711: Healthy Food Choices in Catered Food Situations. APHA Policy Statements 1948-present, cumulative. Washington, DC: APHA, current volume.

- University of Minnesota School of Public Health. Guidelines for Offering Healthy Foods at Meetings, Seminars, and Catered Events. Available at www.ahc.umn. edu/ahc_content/colleges/sph/sph_news/Nutrition.pdf.

- American Cancer Society. 2000. Meeting Well: A Tool for Planning Healthy Meetings and Events. American Cancer Society. www.acsworkplacesolutions.com/ meetingwell.asp.

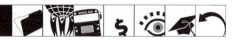
What's in It for Me (WIIFM) is a nutrition awareness, education, and intervention program. Participants log all daily food and beverages consumed as well as daily physical activity for a month. The program increases awareness of the nutritional value of foods as well as energy expenditure. Because weight loss depends on greater caloric or energy expenditure than caloric intake, it is valuable to track this information over time to reach goals of weight loss, weight gain, or weight maintenance.

Goals

- Track average daily nutritional content of foods consumed.
- Track average daily energy expenditure.
- Increase awareness and knowledge of personal energy balance.

Description

Advertise WIIFM by sending out an e-mail asking people to accept the WIIFM nutrition challenge and to attend a one-hour kickoff meeting. WIIFM may be kicked off during a one-hour presentation and discussion session, led by a registered dietitian or nutritionist, on caloric balance and how to estimate caloric intake. The group leader may teach about the benefits of proper nutrition and challenge participants to track their caloric intake for 30 days to learn the content of the foods they are consuming, as well as discover more healthy substitutions that may be lower in calories. The group may meet one time during the kickoff meeting, or weekly for the duration of the program. If the group meets weekly, the registered dietitian or nutritionist may give a presentation and lead a group discussion series on a variety of nutrition topics including healthy recipes and meal preparation. Participants may also discuss their progress, and a question-and-answer period may conclude each session.

Because participants will need to track their daily food and beverage consumption and their daily physical activity, be sure to have food and activity logs available. Many generic logs are available (see the For More Information section), or you can obtain information and quotes on customized nutrition logs from local printers or promotional companies.

Enhancements

- Add cooking demonstrations that provide the caloric value of foods prepared.
- Offer lectures or individual counseling sessions by registered dietitians or nutritionists, exercise physiologists, personal trainers, or health education specialists.
- Provide recipes of the week.
- Provide various exercise options for people at all levels of fitness.
- Pair participants up for social support.
- Provide incentives to anyone who signs up or completes the program. An enrollment incentive may be a personal nutrition journal with a program logo (as described later).
- Provide pre- and postprogram measurements (e.g., body mass index or body composition).

For More Information

- To track your caloric intake and energy expenditure, visit www.mypyramidtracker.gov/.
- Purchase nutrition and fitness logs or journals from a promotional item Web site or local vendor. Journals may be customized by adding the logo of your program or wellness initiative.
- For nutrition education resources, visit www.mypyramid.gov/index.html or www.nutrition.gov/.

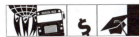
The All You Can Eat board game (available for $39.95 from www.allyoucaneatforkids.com/) is a stand-alone product that teaches basic nutrition knowledge by engaging players to build their breakfast, lunch, and dinner menus while playing a game that is both fun and educational. This program is most appropriate for elementary school students.

Goals

- Increase knowledge about the five food groups and how to eat foods from each of them at every meal.
- Encourage healthy behaviors in children and adults related to eating, sleeping, exercising, and leisure activities.
- Increase knowledge about the importance of balance, variety, and moderation (i.e., portion control) when creating or selecting menus.

Description All You Can Eat, a game of fun and nutrition, engages players with the social activity of menu building. In the process, players come away with a concrete understanding of their own daily nutritional needs. There are 42 healthy lifestyle choice cards and 210 healthy food choice cards in each game. Each player takes a turn by rolling the die and moving a playing piece around the board. Each time a player lands on a colored block, she may select a food item from the corresponding color-coded food cards and record that item on her personal menu. When a player lands on SPIN, she spins the wheel; wherever the arrow stops, she collects at least two food items. Each food item is recorded on a personal menu, which contains slots for each meal: breakfast, lunch, and dinner.

Additionally, while working his way around the board, a player may land on a wild space and pick a wild card. This is a strategic move because sometimes some wild cards allow him to move ahead or spin the wheel. Alternatively, he may select a wild card that causes him to lose a turn because he skipped breakfast or ate too much cake. Included in the wild cards are not only healthy and unhealthy lifestyle lessons but game strategies as well. The first person to complete a menu and cross the finish line is the winner.

The game is bilingual (English and Spanish) and may be played in each language separately, or in both languages simultaneously. This added feature encourages and challenges players to learn other languages, thereby opening the door of opportunity for communication and socialization, not only between English- and Spanish-speaking children, but also among family members and friends.

To integrate the game as part of a health curriculum in schools, teachers may choose to enhance the game with grade-specific curricula designed to teach nutrition from kindergarten through the fifth grade. The curricula offer playing cards for younger audiences that teach fundamental concepts and disciplines to help build a solid foundation for a very young child's nutritional journey through life.

An additional feature to the grade-specific curricula is an audiovisual presentation of the English and Spanish translations of 48 foods from the five food groups as well as translations from the activity books *What is Healthy Living*? and *Healthy Living and More!*

Equipment and Supplies

- One game that may be played with two to four players. You can accommodate more players by creating teams.

>> continued

- Grade-specific curricula may be purchased separately. Included in the curricula are grade-specific activities, coloring pages, word searches, food group tracking sheets, and English and Spanish audiovisual translations. The cost per grade or per classroom varies based on the quantity purchased at $250 each. All worksheets are reproducible.

- A DVD player is needed to play a bilingual video that demonstrates how the game is played and provides bilingual translations that complement the curriculum.

- Pencils, crayons, or markers for menu recording.

Enhancements

- The greatest enhancement to this game is the curriculum. Included in the curriculum are English and Spanish translations, an instructional video on how to play, coloring books that tell nutrition stories, word games, puzzles, worksheets, and food tracking sheets.

- A very simple enhancement that may be implemented as part of a classroom lesson is to offer a reward system for participation in game-related question and answer sessions. Reward tracking sheets are an added feature to help encourage participation by placing stickers or stars on each child's sheet. Rewards may be as simple as non-food-related class privileges. A reward tracking sheet may be as simple as a piece of paper with the child's name on it.

- Institute challenges using the take-home tracking sheets, included in the curriculum, which may be both fun and competitive and encourage family accountability.

- Engage parents by encouraging children to teach their parents about nutrition.

For More Information   Visit http:///www.allyoucaneatforkids.com/.

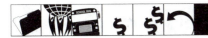

Healthy Eating Every Day helps adults make nutrition and lifestyle changes that will have a positive impact on their lives. There are fees associated with this program; each participant must pay $34.95 for a participant package (bulk discounts apply), and the facilitator must pay $364 for facilitator training.

Goals

- Help people improve their health and quality of life by teaching proven behavior change strategies.
- Teach appropriate lifestyle skills, based on an evidence-based, readiness to change model.
- Assist adults in meeting federal nutrition guidelines.

Description

Healthy Eating Every Day teaches participants how to choose the proper balance of the right foods for optimal health, set realistic goals and rewards, and cope with triggers for unhealthy eating. They also learn to consider healthy eating while shopping for food, eat well when dining out, and make sense of nutrition information—all without having to eliminate entire food groups or sacrifice meals. The information is in line with and complements the USDA nutrition guidelines.

Many organizations use Healthy Eating Every Day to empower people to change their health habits. Classes may be taught in person, online, or in combination; either in groups or with individuals; and in 14 or 20 weeks. Most in-person classes meet once a week for about one hour; online classes vary. The success the program has had in these varied settings may be traced to the following:

- **Proven effectiveness.** Healthy Eating Every Day was developed in partnership with The Cooper Institute, which has achieved worldwide recognition for its outstanding scientific research, and has been proven effective in clinical trials.
- **Structure and support.** The program structure builds a strong foundation of behavior change and a community of support, which helps entrench individual wellness habits.
- **Inclusive approach.** Participants build on small successes to create confidence. This method appeals to even people who are just starting on their journey to better health.
- **Personalized strategies.** The course allows participants to tailor the program based on their readiness to change, lifestyle, and preferences so each person gets the information needed to reach his or her health and nutrition goals and make lasting changes.

Equipment and Supplies

- Facilitator package (includes a binder, CD-ROM, online course, and Web site resources)
- Participant package for each person who takes the course (includes a book, online course, and Web site resources)
- Food models (optional)

Enhancements

- Schedule tours to local areas of interest, such as grocery stores or farmers markets.
- Invite guest speakers to offer additional information based on program topics.
- Provide a healthy snack during class to introduce participants to new foods and to demonstrate portion sizes.

For More Information

Visit www.activeliving.info; call 800-747-4457; or send an e-mail to alpinfo@hkusa.com.

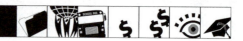

Veggin' Out is a nutrition awareness and education program that may be implemented in worksite, community, and school settings. This award-winning program educates participants about the health benefits of eating fruits and vegetables. It provides education on healthy ways to select, prepare, cook, and store fruits and vegetables through live cooking demonstrations and the distribution of recipe cards. Chefs certified in food safety conduct cooking demonstrations for the audience with interactive teaching techniques.

Goals

- Increase fruit and vegetable consumption by providing information on the many health benefits of a diet high in fruits and vegetables.
- Increase knowledge and skills related to the proper selection, preparation, cooking, and storage of fruits and vegetables.

Description

Two chefs stand behind a colorful table dicing, slicing, cooking, educating, and entertaining inner-city elementary school students at an after-school community center. "What is this vegetable?" the chef asks the children. "Asparagus!" a child shouts out, surprising the chefs. "Terrific!" responds the chef. "How about this one? Do you know what this vegetable is?" "Broccoli!" the children say in unison. The cooking demonstration and the interactive education continue for about 30 minutes until stir-fried vegetable samples are ready to be distributed to the audience.

Johnson & Wales' Veggin' Out program demonstrates culturally diverse and nutritious recipes that incorporate fresh, locally grown, in-season produce. The Johnson & Wales chefs cook behind an attractive display on hot plates in their chef uniforms. The table is covered with a white cloth, and colorful, fresh fruits and vegetables head the table. The program is engaging, interactive, educational, and fun! The Veggin' Out logo is cartoon-like, colorful, and eye-catching to children of all ages.

You may offer a similar program at your worksite, in your community, or at your school by contacting your local culinary college, or any college in your area that offers a culinary arts program. Students or staff may be willing to do creative cooking demonstrations. Your employees may also have culinary skills that they may be willing to share. Employees at one hospital were surprised to learn that the director of emergency management was a chef who operated a part-time catering business. He provided cooking demonstrations with fresh vegetables at the hospital's health fair at no charge. The hospital gave scheduled time off for employees to attend.

Enhancements

- Provide take-home recipes.
- Use this program to kick off the Community Cookbook program.
- Offer the program for four consecutive weeks if you have food safety–certified chefs available.
- Add this demonstration to health fairs, farmers markets, or other wellness events.

For More Information

Contact the Feinstein Community Service Center, Johnson & Wales University, at 401-598-2989 or e-mail feinsteincenter@jwu.edu., or contact a culinary arts school in your area.

General Health and Prevention Programs

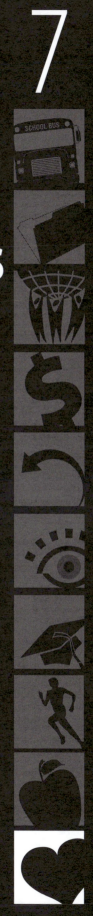

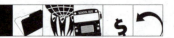
15 for 15 is a 15-minute chair massage program that costs $15 per person. This program may be implemented at worksites, in schools, or in a variety of community locations such as malls, fire stations, police stations, and senior centers. It is designed to provide relief for both physical and mental stress symptoms. Chair massage may be performed in facility lobbies or in small private rooms.

Goals

- Reduce stress.
- Improve circulation.

Description

Travelers just stop by, without an appointment, in the airport terminal and enjoy a quick massage to reduce their stress. Workers may sign up in advance for a weekly chair massage at their worksite. A chiropractor may encourage patients to have a 15-minute on-site massage after treatment on a specific area of the body. After a cold and rigorous day on the slopes, skiers may stop by the lodge for a chair massage. After a tough workout, health club members may get a quick massage in the lobby of the health club on their way out the door.

These are just a few of the many situations in which chair massage is being offered. Offering a quick, low-cost massage at a convenient location reduces the barriers of time and money and increases engagement in stress reduction programs. Sometimes even having to make an appointment may cause stress. On-site services with no advance appointments required may provide a solution for those with tight schedules. Just 15 minutes of massage to the neck, back, arms, and hands may decrease circulatory problems common in office workers and improve energy levels while providing a much-appreciated break for employees.

To find massage therapists, consider the following:

- Contact local massage therapists to see if they are willing to offer their services on site. Organizations or participants may pay massage therapists directly. Organizations may require a percentage of the therapist's total revenue for the use of space and marketing fees. Ask for proof of liability insurance.
- Contact massage therapy schools. Many massage students have hands-on patient treatment requirements they need to fulfill. It is possible to have a massage student on site for free for a limited period of time. Consult with an attorney regarding liability issues.

Enhancements

- Add this program prior to or after an educational workshop or lecture.
- Distribute educational handouts on the benefits of massage and stress reduction strategies.
- Provide weekly sessions such as on every Monday.
- Add massage to other events such as health fairs or Stress-Less Day.
- Employers may cover the cost of a massage therapist one day per week as a benefit or incentive for employees.

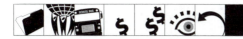

Laugh It Up! is a one-hour program designed to improve mood and reduce stress. A building body of research indicates that laughter also improves health. Laugh It Up! may be implemented by hiring local comedians, posting or e-mailing weekly jokes, or showing humorous movies.

Goals

- Improve mood.
- Reduce stress.
- Improve overall health.

Description   "The old saying 'laughter is the best medicine' appears to be true when it comes to protecting your heart," reports Michael Miller, MD, director of the Center for Preventive Cardiology at the University of Maryland Medical Center. "We don't know yet why laughing protects the heart, but we do know that mental stress is associated with impairment of the endothelium, the protective barrier lining our blood vessels. This can cause a series of inflammatory reactions that lead to fat and cholesterol build-up in the coronary arteries and ultimately, to a heart attack" (www.umm.edu/features/laughter.htm).

Schedule four different one-hour weekly Laugh It Up! activities. You can show a comedy film the first week, and arrange for a local comedian to perform the second week (contact a local comedian, or advertise within your organization in case you have your own in-house comedian). On the third week, invite participants to bring their favorite jokes or comics to share. The last week could involve participants listening to a funny story or CD or watching another comedy film (rent or purchase comedy movies, joke books, and comic books).

Enhancement   Give a workshop or presentation on the benefits of laughter.

For More Information   Visit www.umm.edu/features/laughter.htm.

Stop, Stretch, and Breathe
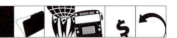

Stop, Stretch, and Breathe is a 10-minute stress management and physical activity performed in a chair. This program may be offered at worksites, community-based organizations, or schools prior to meetings, classes, or workshops, or as a stand-alone program. Stop, Stretch, and Breathe may be offered as an eight-week series or as an ongoing program.

Goals

- Increase blood flow and improve range of motion through stretching.
- Reduce stress through muscle relaxation and deep breathing.

Description

You may immediately identify the smell of lavender when you enter the room for your Stop, Stretch, and Breathe class. The sound of water is coming from a small waterfall on a table in the front of the room. The lights are dim, and a screen saver of a fish tank is projected from a laptop computer on the front wall of the room. Ocean sounds emanate from a softly playing CD. All of these staging techniques help to enhance relaxation. The instructor, standing at the entrance to the room, encourages you to take a seat and begin to unwind for a few moments before the session begins.

Begin the session by walking participants through the following steps:

1. Sit up straight and maintain this posture. Let your head balance between your shoulders so you feel no strain in your neck.
2. Close your eyes if you feel comfortable enough to do so. (If not, ask participants to focus their attention on the fish tank screen saver or other relaxing visual projected on the front wall of the room.)
3. Clear your mind, letting go of any stressful, negative, or judging thoughts.
4. Notice your breathing. Your breathing should be slow and fairly regular, without any big gulps of air. Notice your chest rising and falling. Notice the feeling of air entering and exiting your throat.
5. Notice any tightness, soreness, or stiffness in your muscles. Try to relax these muscles by tensing and relaxing them. Notice the difference between tension and relaxation.

Demonstrate and perform the following exercises (and be sure to have copies of this list to hand out):

1. Do five repetitions of each of the following:
   - Deep, relaxing breaths
   - Forward neck rolls
   - Front shoulder rolls
   - Back shoulder rolls
   - Upward shoulder shrugs while breathing in, and shoulder drops when breathing out
   - Shoulder retractions by pulling the shoulders back so that the shoulder blades move toward each other

2. Deeply inhale while raising both arms above your head. Hold for a moment then gradually lower your arms while slowly exhaling.

3. Raise one arm, bend to the side, and lower the arm slowly. Repeat with the other arm.

4. Raise your arms over your head again, and this time fold forward slowly, lowering your head between your legs until the top of your head faces toward the floor. Hold this position for several seconds while continuing to breathe. (This exercise is similar to inverted poses in yoga.)

5. With your hands on your thighs just above your kneecaps, come up *very* slowly with your back in an arched (i.e., cat stretch) position.

6. Return to a seated position and resume a straight posture.

7. Notice whether any muscles in your body are still tense. If so, tense and relax those muscles until all strain is gone.

8. End the session with five deep, relaxing breaths.

Enhancements

- Add more chair yoga exercises, such as the seated triangle pose, to extend the length of the program.

- Provide educational materials on stress management.

- Add a 10-minute educational component, or pair with an educational lecture provided by a health care professional or vendor (e.g., employee assistance program).

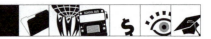

Stress-Less Day is a one-day stress management event that is both an awareness and educational program. It may be offered in worksite, community, and school settings, and may be creatively enhanced in a variety of ways. According to the National Institute for Occupational Safety and Health, one-fourth of employees view their jobs as the number one stressor in their lives. Health care expenditures are nearly 50 percent greater for workers who report high levels of stress. Stress is associated with poor health, injury, increased absenteeism, tardiness, and intentions by workers to quit their jobs. Faculty, teachers, and students are also under a high degree of stress as a result of increases in academic performance standards and family pressures. During these tough financial times, communities are also struggling with significant budget cuts and their consequences.

Goals

- Increase awareness of the negative effects of stress.
- Increase knowledge and skills to prevent, cope with, and reduce stress through positive health behaviors, practices, and programs.

Description   When employees at the state health department entered the main conference room where large meetings were usually held, they felt as though they were being transported to another place. One employee described the experience of entering the room as "entering a tranquil paradise, far, far away from work." The room they once knew as a typical conference room was totally transformed! For a short time, employees felt as though they were not in the same building. The conference room now had dim lighting, candles that gave a soft glow around the room, the smell of hot apple cider, and the faint sound of ocean tides. All of the employees' senses were engaged, resulting in an immediate reduction in stress before participating in any program activities. This one-day program ran from 10:00 a.m. to 4:00 p.m., allowing employees to stop by at their convenience. Registration or appointments were not required. Employees could participate as long and as frequently as they wanted throughout the course of the day. No requirements. No expectations. No stress!

Developed by the Rhode Island Department of Health in collaboration with the state employee wellness initiative, Get Fit, Rhode Island!, Stress-Less Day became an award-winning program by providing education and increasing the awareness of stress prevention and reduction. This program was offered to state employees a few weeks prior to the holiday season when program participation is typically low. However, more than one-third of all employees in the department attended this event! Employees reported on a health interest survey (discussed in chapter 2) that this was the time of year they struggled with finding a balance between work and family or personal life because of elevated stress levels.

You may incorporate several program offerings into Stress-Less Day. Be sure you've secured people to assist with these program offerings:

- Massage. Contact a local massage school to find practitioners who could provide free five-minute chair or hand massages under a small tent to provide a cozy experience.
- Hot drinks. Everyone likes a hot drink with a relaxing aroma in the winter. Provide samples of apple cider from a crock pot. Hot tea or hot chocolate are other options.

- Atmosphere. Use staging techniques from chapter 3 to create a relaxing atmosphere. Provide dim lighting with lamps and candles (no fluorescent lighting). Play soft, relaxing background music. Set up overhead tents in the room to provide a comfortable atmosphere. Tablecloths, fresh flowers, and tabletop waterfalls add that special touch for optimal relaxation.

- Employee assistance. If you have an employee assistance program, now is the time to bring in program representatives. Stress-Less Day provides an opportunity for representatives to casually chat with employees and set up appointments.

- Educational materials. At an educational table, provide handouts and information on healthy coping skills and strategies to prevent or reduce holiday-related stress as well as year-round stress.

- Gift wrapping. If your program is being held during the holiday season, invite each employee to bring in one holiday gift to be wrapped free of charge. Provide last-minute lists of great gift ideas for items under $20.

- Yoga and meditation. Provide yoga and meditation demonstrations every half hour throughout the day. Provide handouts on techniques so participants can practice at home and in their work spaces.

Enhancements

- Offer Stress-Less Day every week between Thanksgiving and New Year's Day.

- Expand the number of stress-related lectures, workshops, and demonstrations to other conference rooms or locations.

- In schools, offer stress-less activities at the end of the school day so family members may participate when they arrive to pick up their children.

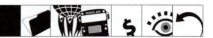

Musical Happy Hour is a musical therapy program designed to reduce stress, increase motivation to exercise, and increase physical activity. Musical Happy Hour helps workers wind down from the week and offers them an opportunity to socialize and enrich their lives by listening to live classical music. Music has also been shown to enhance physical performance. Participants in exercise programs often report increased motivation and enhanced physical activity performance during and after listening to music.

Goals

- Reduce stress.
- Increase motivation to exercise.
- Increase physical activity.

Description

To reduce afternoon commuter traffic, a city offers workers a Musical Happy Hour. Commuters gather on Friday nights to listen to classical music and enjoy a cool or hot seasonal beverage with healthy snacks for an hour of unwinding prior to battling traffic out of the city. To reduce the number of people leaving the city at the same time, adding to already heavy commuter traffic, this program helps workers reduce stress before starting out on what may be a long journey home to their families.

The cost of this program can be minimal if you can arrange for a live band to volunteer or play CDs on a high-quality sound system. (Be sure you've secured a space with adequate seating.) You may have contacts through a member of your organization, or know of a local band that would volunteer for publicity. A potluck of healthy snacks may be offered, or fresh fruits may be donated by local farmers or specialty grocers looking to advertise their products. Invite people to sign up so you can plan for attendance and food or you can allow walk-ins.

Enhancements

- Offer Musical Happy Hour during the workday or school day. The program may be particularly effective during high stress times for people in the organization (e.g., tax season for an accounting firm, final exams for students).

- Music can also enhance motivation to exercise and improve exercise performance. If promoting physical activity, encourage participants to create a list of music selections that motivate them or charge them up. Through a habitual response, participants may experience an increase in motivation to exercise simply by hearing their favorite music.

- You can incorporate music to promote physical and emotional well-being in many situations. Be creative and look for opportunities to energize your participants with music!

- Senior centers, senior housing facilities, and nursing homes may offer Musical Happy Hour with coffee or tea and play music from the era of participants' youth to improve mood and reduce stress.

- Offer opportunities for physical activity during Musical Happy Hour.

- Add dance instruction to physical activity offerings.

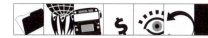

Pet Therapy

Pet Therapy is a program that may be implemented in worksite, community, or school settings. Domestic pets have been shown to improve mood, reduce stress, increase physical activity, and in some studies, improve both psychological well-being and physical health.

Goals

- Improve mood.
- Reduce stress.
- Increase physical activity.
- Improve psychological well-being.
- Improve physical health.

Description

Pet Therapy is a stress management program that may be offered in a variety of settings by inviting employees, community members, or students to bring a pet to work, community gatherings, or school, or by hiring a certified pet therapist. (You can also contact a local pet store or animal shelter to see whether they would be able to visit your organization with pets.) Pets may visit room to room at worksites, schools, hospitals, or other community-based organizations, or they may be supervised in a room where people may visit to take a stress break. The length and frequency of the program may vary from a one-time, or annual, all-day Pet Therapy Day or Bring Your Pet to Work Day to a weekly one-hour Pet Therapy program with an individual or a small group.

Note: To ensure the health of participants and pets alike, pet owners should provide proof of rabies and other vaccinations prior to enrolling their pets in the program.

Many research studies have confirmed the positive health benefits pets provide. The therapeutic use of pets as companions has gained increasing attention in recent years for a wide variety of patients—people with AIDS or cancer, the elderly, and the developmentally disabled. Animals provide a constant source of comfort and focus for attention. Some of us have heard stories of a cat sitting on the bed of a dying resident, knowing when the resident was about to pass, and providing company and comfort in the person's time of need. They bring out our nurturing instinct and make us feel safe and unconditionally accepted. Certified pet therapists are trained to provide pet therapy with pets that are vaccinated, docile, and well trained.

Enhancements

- In residential facilities, walking with pets may also improve physical activity, even if Pet Therapy simply encourages residents to walk down hallways.
- Worksites may offer Pet Therapy Day or Bring Your Pet to Work Day, during which employees may go out and walk their dogs together while getting physical activity themselves.

For More Information

Visit www.activitytherapy.com/national.htm.

Kick Colds and Flu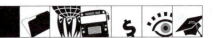

Kick Colds and Flu is a low cost, easy-to-implement educational program on proper hand-washing techniques designed to prevent or reduce the spread of germs, particularly during the colder months of the year when people may be more susceptible to the common cold and flu.

Goals

- Improve preventive self-care behaviors.
- Reduce the spread of the common cold and flu.

Description

The Kick Colds and Flu program increases awareness by providing education on the importance and benefits of proper hand washing. According to the U.S. Centers for Disease Control and Prevention (CDC), proper hand washing is the number one preventive measure we can take to avoid getting colds and flu. CDC recommends the following steps for proper hand washing:

- Wash hands using soap and warm, running water.
- Rub the hands vigorously during washing for at least 20 seconds. Pay special attention to the backs of the hands, the wrists, between the fingers, and under the fingernails.
- Rinse the hands well while leaving the water running.
- With the water running, dry the hands with a single-use towel.
- Turn off the water using a paper towel, covering washed hands to prevent recontamination.

Although most people report washing their hands frequently, many do not wash them thoroughly enough to eliminate all germs. As a result, germs may still be spread from one person to another. People may not wash their hands long enough or may not know proper hand-washing procedures. Therefore, providing information or education on this topic is critical for the prevention and control of colds and flu, particularly during flu season or the colder months of the year, and in certain environments (day care).

Kick Colds and Flu is a stop-by program designed to conveniently increase awareness of and provide education on proper hand-washing techniques. A table is set up in a highly visible, high-traffic location with a display board providing information on cold and flu prevention. Glo Germ is an easy-to-use, low-cost product that may be used for live, interactive demonstrations of proper hand-washing techniques.

When a participant visits the Kick Colds and Flu display table or booth, the educator provides her with Glo Germ lotion to thoroughly rub on her hands. The participant is then requested to wash her hands, as she normally would, at a nearby sink and return to the booth. When the participant returns, the educator places an ultraviolet light over the participant's hands to reveal any residue lotion, indicating where germs are still present on her hands. Mr. Joe Kingsley, president of Glo Germ, reports that demonstrations with this product have been very effective in increasing the awareness of sanitary practices among elementary and middle school students. "The children love the interactive demonstration. School nurses and teachers report the information is being retained long past the demonstrations."

Equipment and Supplies

- Glo Germ lotion
- Ultraviolet lamp
- Table
- Display board
- Educational handouts

Enhancements

- Give away sample hand sanitizers.
- Provide a raffle for participants to win prizes.
- Combine Kick Colds and Flu with a flu shot clinic.

For More Information   Call 800-842-6622 or visit www.glogerm.com. You can also purchase Glo Germ lotions from this site. The cost of this program ranges from $10 to $110.

Breast Health for Seniors

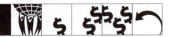

Breast Health for Seniors is an innovative and award-winning program for older women that addresses their concerns regarding mammography, eliminating barriers and encouraging screening.

Goals

- Promote breast cancer screening.
- Increase the number of older women who are having mammograms.
- Educate older women about breast cancer and the myths and facts surrounding it.

Description

Breast Health for Seniors reaches out to women over the age of 60. This program is held at community senior centers and senior housing developments. It includes a short informational presentation on breast cancer and mammography by a health educator. The discussion includes mammography issues and concerns, Medicare coverage, and personal experiences. Usually a breast cancer survivor shares her own experience. In addition, arrangements are made with a local mammography center to send a representative who can describe the procedure and schedule a mammography appointment at the event. As an added incentive, a $15 gift certificate to a local restaurant, which offsets the Medicare mammography co-payment of $17, is provided to any woman who schedules her mammogram at the event. The health educator also leads the attendees in making breast cancer awareness bracelets for themselves, family members, and friends.

The cost of this program can vary, depending on the number of participants and whether you order the Breast Health for Seniors PowerPoint presentation kit (contact information is provided later).

Equipment and Supplies

- Breast Health for Seniors PowerPoint presentation kit (available for $25)
- Laptop computer, LCD projector, and screen
- Printed educational material on breast cancer
- $15 gift certificates to local restaurants
- Pink and white or clear beads, cancer awareness ribbon charms, jewelry thread, Super Glue, and scissors
- Promotional materials such as flyers and posters

Enhancements

- Set up a breast cancer information table to include giveaway materials on treatment options, support groups, and screening guidelines.
- Invite local breast cancer advocacy groups to participate.
- Invite local high school students to assist with the program and motivate attendees.

For More Information

- For the Breast Health for Seniors PowerPoint presentation kit or breast cancer educational materials, contact the Rhode Island Cancer Council at 866-879-4100 (toll free) or 401-728-4800 for more details and assistance, or visit www.ricancercouncil.org/index.php.
- Breast Health for Seniors will be published in the *Journal of Cancer Education*, and you can read the article for more information (Glicksman et al., in press).

PawSox and Prostates is an innovative and award-winning program designed to encourage men, particularly those who are Hispanic or African American (ethnicities identified at highest risk for prostate cancer), as well as socioeconomically depressed populations, to be screened for prostate cancer. Held at a local minor league baseball stadium, the PawSox stadium, the program is in a setting comfortable for men. The program is presented by male physicians and the prostate-specific antigen (PSA) blood test for prostate cancer screening is available free of charge that evening, provided by a local hospital.

Goals

- Promote prostate cancer screening in high-risk populations.
- Increase the number of men who are screened for prostate cancer.
- Educate men about prostate cancer, screening methods, and treatment options.

Description

PawSox and Prostates reaches out to men over the age of 40. This program is held at a local minor league baseball stadium; PawSox stadium. The program includes two tickets to the baseball game, a barbecue buffet, and a short informational presentation on prostate cancer by local urologists and oncologists. The discussion includes information on prostate cancer, screening (PSA blood test and digital rectal examination), treatment options, and other concerns. In addition, arrangements are made with a local hospital for on-site phlebotomists to draw blood samples from participants for PSA testing. Blood samples are then sent to a clinical laboratory for analysis. Following the event, participants are notified of their results in one of the following three ways: 1) If participants have indicated a primary physician, the results are sent by the local hospital to these physicians as well as to the participants; 2) If participants have not indicated a primary physician, the local hospital will contact the participant to give them the results and to also try to get them into a health care practice; or 3) If participants have an elevated PSA, the local hospital provides free follow-up services if the participant has no insurance and no primary physician. To tailor this event to your community, contact representatives of a local baseball stadium or minor league baseball team to make arrangements and consider renaming the program in such a way that it fits with your local athletic team.

Equipment and Supplies

- Tickets to a baseball game and barbecue
- Private area for blood drawing by local hospital phlebotomists to protect patient privacy
- Printed educational material on prostate cancer
- Promotional materials such as flyers and posters

Enhancements

- Make arrangements for local urologists, medical oncologist(s), and radiation oncologist(s) to present information and to provide individual consultation.
- Make arrangements for a local hospital chaplain or social worker to provide individual consultation.

>> continued

- Set up a prostate cancer information table to include giveaway materials on treatment options, support groups, and screening guidelines.
- Invite local cancer advocacy groups to participate.
- Provide giveaways.

For More Information

- For prostate cancer educational materials (for a low fee), contact the Rhode Island Cancer Council at 866-879-4100 (toll free) or 401-728-4800 for more details and assistance, or visit www.ricancercouncil.org/index.php.

- Free or low-cost information and educational materials on prostate cancer are also available from the National Cancer Institute's Cancer Information Service at 800-4-CANCER (800-422-6237) or TTY:800-332-8615 (toll free) or visit www.cancer.gov/.

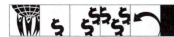

Sun Smarts is a skin cancer prevention program designed to screen people for skin cancer at local beaches, provide information and educational materials, encourage people to use sunscreen, provide skin examinations by dermatology residents, and refer participants for further testing when necessary. The cost may be kept low if the event is sponsored by community-based agencies. The cost may be high if you advertise the event on radio or television stations.

Goals

- Promote regular skin screenings, particularly to populations with high sun exposure.
- Promote sun safety.
- Educate beachgoers about skin cancer.

Description

Sun Smarts is a skin cancer prevention program that reaches out to all populations in a location where sun exposure is high. This program is held at local beaches (be sure to contact your state department of environmental management for permission to hold your program at a local beach). The program includes cancer educational materials and a free skin examination by local dermatology residents or dermatologists. In addition, arrangements can be made with a local television station to provide a media campaign and equipment.

Equipment and Supplies

- Registration table with chairs
- Covered or tented waiting area with chairs
- Covered or tented examination area with privacy screens and chairs
- Registration forms for recording of skin abnormalities
- Printed educational material on skin cancer and sun safety, including coloring books for children
- Giveaways (e.g., sunscreen samples, water bottles)

Enhancements

- Make arrangements for nurses to review noted skin abnormalities and make physician referrals.
- Set up a skin cancer information table.
- Promote the event to local television or radio stations for media coverage (i.e., during weather reports).

For More Information

- For skin cancer educational materials and coloring books (for a low fee), contact the Rhode Island Cancer Council at 866-879-4100 (toll free) or 401-728-4800 for more details and assistance, or visit www.ricancercouncil.org/index.php.
- Free or low-cost information and educational materials on skin cancer are also available from the National Cancer Institute's Cancer Information Service at 800-4-CANCER (800-422-6237) or TTY:800-332-8615 (toll free), or visit www.cancer.gov/.

Colossal Colon

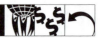

The Colossal Colon is a 40-foot-long (12 m), 4-foot-tall (1.2 m), crawl-through model of the human colon complete with polyps and various diseases of the colon and stages of colorectal cancer. Adults and children alike may crawl through or look through windows for a visual or hands-on learning experience about Crohn's disease, diverticular disease, ulcerative colitis, hemorrhoids, cancerous and noncancerous polyps, and various stages of colon cancer.

Goals

- Increase awareness of colon and colorectal cancer.
- Educate the public on the importance of colorectal cancer screening.

Description

After being diagnosed with colon cancer on her 23rd birthday, Molly McMaster wanted to tell the world that anyone could get the disease. Her first crazy project, Rolling to Recovery, was a 2,000-mile (3,219 km) journey on inline skates from New York to Colorado, during which she got an e-mail from a young woman in Little Rock, Arkansas, named Amanda Sherwood Roberts. Amanda had been diagnosed with the disease at 24 years of age, and the two young women became immediate friends. Eventually, Amanda nominated Molly to carry the 2002 Salt Lake Olympic Torch, and after Molly was chosen, the two women finally got the chance to meet in person and tell their story to Katie Couric on the *Today* show. After the show, Katie told Molly, "If you come up with anything crazy for Colorectal Cancer Awareness Month (March), let us know. We'll have you back on the show!" The wheels began to turn in Molly's head . . . .

On December 30, 2002, Molly carried the Olympic Torch through Saratoga Springs, New York. Amanda died just two days later at her home in Little Rock at the age of 27. Along with Amanda's cousin, Hannah Vogler, Molly decided that she needed to do something in honor of her friend. Together the two girls built the Colossal Colon, affectionately known as Coco. Since 2002, Coco has visited over 100 cities in over 40 states and Canada, and has been hosted at hospitals, malls, convention centers, state fairs, museums, a football tournament, an amusement park, and other unique locations.

The Colossal Colon may be rented for display at your worksite, community-based organization, or school. The cost depends on the shipping distance. Basic rental requirements for the Colossal Colon are as follows:

- Rental of the Colossal Colon for up to one week
- Transportation (trucking) to get the Colossal Colon to your site
- A supervisor to help you set up and break down the Colossal Colon correctly
- Colossal Colon brochures including general information about colorectal cancer
- A storyboard telling the story of the Colossal Colon
- A sign listing the symptoms of colorectal cancer
- A B-roll video and high-quality digital photographs of the Colossal Colon for use in press releases, public service announcements, and advertising

To accommodate the Colossal Colon, your hosting site must have an entrance the size of double doors. Because the Colossal Colon takes up a space of approximately 20 by 20 feet (6 by 6 m), a space of least 40 by 40 feet (12 by 12 m) is recommended. The site must be either indoors or under a 40-by-40-foot tent with solid flooring. Labor is needed for unloading and loading the Colossal Colon, and volunteers or labor is needed for staffing the Colossal Colon while it is open to visitors. Although media materials are available as part of the rental agreement, the hosting organization is responsible for arranging for any advertising and publicity surrounding the event. Visit www.youtube.com/watch?v=8H5FdrBVotc for a virtual tour of the Colossal Colon.

Enhancements

- Arrange for a colorectal cancer survivor or survivors to speak at the event.
- Provide multilingual handouts and educational materials on colorectal cancer prevention, diagnosis, and treatment.
- Partner with multilingual health care professionals from local hospitals and gastrointestinal clinics to answer questions and offer on-site bookings for colonoscopies.
- Offer incentives to people who follow up with colorectal cancer screening.
- Include the exhibit as part of a comprehensive health fair.

For More Information   Visit www.colonclub.com/colossalcolon.html.

Pink Spirit Week

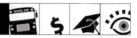

Pink Spirit Week is a breast cancer education initiative directed toward high school students to teach them about breast cancer, risk reduction, detection methods, and treatment. (This program is also appropriate for college and university students.) The information is presented in health education classes or at an assembly by a local oncologist or health educator. This program is three pronged: (1) breast cancer education, (2) Pink *Spirit* to garner enthusiasm among the students via athletics, and (3) community involvement.

Goals

- Educate high school students about all facets of breast cancer.
- Educate family members and friends via the students.
- Promote breast cancer awareness and advocacy.

Description   Pink Spirit Week reaches out to all high schools to promote breast cancer education. This program is held at participating high schools through health education classes or in an assembly. Local oncology medical professionals or health educators teach the classes using PowerPoint presentations. A breast cancer survivor shares her story for personal impact. Students are given pink ribbons (pins and stickers) to wear during this week. Permission is requested from the local interscholastic league to allow athletes and referees to wear pink terry-cloth wristbands at sporting events. Schools are given freedom to encourage Pink Spirit through other activities such as a Dress Down Day or Wear Pink Day. To extend the program into the greater community, students are encouraged to participate in breast cancer awareness programs throughout the state, or to plan and present a fund-raising event to pay for the program.

Equipment and Supplies

Education Component

- PowerPoint presentation kit on breast cancer awareness (available for $25)
- Laptop, LCD projector, and screen
- Printed educational material on breast cancer, including material designed for teens and men

Spirit Component

- Pink ribbons
- Pink terry-cloth wristbands

Community Component   Equipment and supply needs vary with the choice of activity.

Enhancements

- Ask a breast cancer survivor to share her story.
- Demonstrate breast self-examination using models (teen model preferred).
- Play Myths and Facts game with prizes for winners.
- Involve a local or state representative.
- Invite local breast cancer advocacy groups to participate.

For More Information   For the Pink Spirit PowerPoint presentation kit or breast cancer educational materials, contact the Rhode Island Cancer Council at 866-879-4100 (toll free) or 401-728-4800 for more details and assistance, or visit www.ricancercouncil.org/index.php.

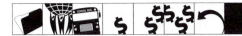

A customized health risk intervention (HRI) starts the health behavior change process by pinpointing each participant's stage of change for each health risk and delivering targeted guidance on the most important steps to take to start progressing. The HRI is then followed by computerized, tailored LifeStyle Management programs to help participants make needed behavior changes in the areas of smoking, stress management, weight management, regular exercise, depression prevention, and medication adherence. There is a fee of $35 per person per year for this program. Access the program at www.prochange.com/products.

Goals

- Apply the best that the science of health behavior change has to offer participants at each stage of change.
- Move those in the precontemplation (not ready), contemplation (getting ready), and preparation (ready) stages, to the action (making the behavior change) and maintenance (sustaining the behavior change) stages.

Description   Pro-Change's LifeStyle Management programs include two carefully targeted components: computerized, tailored interventions and interactive stage-matched e-workbooks. The seven LifeStyle programs use statistical decision making to create individualized paths for change for each participant and deliver the guidance each participant is ready to apply. Each time a participant returns to the program, he receives feedback on how he is doing, what change strategies he is using well and which he may be underusing, and what steps he can take to make progress. The programs are complemented by interactive, stage-matched e-workbooks that help keep participants on track with guidance and inspiration. All seven of the programs produced significant results in clinical trials with large populations. Participants need Internet access to take part in this program.

Enhancements

- The Proactive Health Consumer program module may be added to the LifeStyle suite.
- Adult Responsible Drinking, Healthy Eating, and Financial Well-Being programs may be added as well.

For More Information   To find additional information about implementing any of the Pro-Change programs, or to view a short demo of one LifeStyle program, go to www.prochange.com/stressdemo, or contact Janice M. Prochaska, PhD, at 401-874-4109 or jmprochaska@prochange.com.

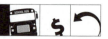

The U.S. Centers for Disease Control and Prevention (CDC) developed the School Health Index, a self-assessment and planning guide that may be used as part of a comprehensive school health improvement program. Promoting healthy and safe behaviors among students is an important part of the fundamental mission of schools: to provide young people with the knowledge and skills to become healthy and productive adults. By promoting health and safety, schools can increase students' capacity to learn, reduce absences, and improve physical fitness and mental alertness. The School Health Index is available at no cost and may be implemented in as little as six hours. This program is most appropriate for elementary through high school settings.

Goals

- Identify the strengths and weaknesses of your school's health and safety policies and programs.
- Develop an action plan for improving student health.
- Involve teachers, parents, students, and the community in improving school policies and programs.

Description   The School Health Index provides structure and direction to schools' efforts to improve health and safety policies and programs. First released in 2000, the School Health Index has been used by schools in nearly every state in the United States and in Canada. It is designed for use at the local level. However, with appropriate adaptation, it may be used at the district level as well, especially if the district has only a few schools and those schools have similar policies and programs.

The health and safety habits of students are influenced by the entire school environment. Therefore, the School Health Index has eight modules, each corresponding to a component of a coordinated school health program:

- Health education
- Physical education
- Health services
- Nutrition services

- Counseling
- Healthy school environment
- Health promotion for staff
- Family and community involvement

A team of representatives from various groups within your school—parents, teachers, students, administrators, other staff members, and concerned community members—is responsible for completing eight self-assessment modules. Responses to the items are scored to help you identify your school's strengths and weaknesses. The School Health Index includes a Planning for Improvement section to help your school develop an action plan for improving student health. The results from the School Health Index may help you include health promotion activities in your overall School Improvement Plan, which will ultimately allow you to develop an ongoing process for monitoring progress and reviewing your recommendations for change. The School Health Index is *your* school's self-assessment tool, and it should not be used to compare schools or evaluate the staff. There is no such thing as a passing grade on the School Health Index. You should use your scores only to help you understand your school's strengths and weaknesses and to develop an action plan for improving the promotion and management of health and safety.

Many of the improvements that you may want to make after completing the School Health Index may be done with your existing staff and resources. For those priority actions that do require additional resources, the results may stimulate school board and community support for school health programs. A small investment of time may pay big dividends in improving students' well-being, readiness to learn, and prospects for a healthy life.

Enhancements

- The fourth edition of the School Health Index addresses behaviors that play a critical role in preventing the leading causes of death, disability, hospitalization, and illness among young people and adults in the United States:
  - Physical activity and physical education
  - Nutrition
  - Tobacco use prevention
  - Unintentional injury and violence prevention
  - Asthma
- Future editions also will address other health issues that have a major impact on the current and future health of young people, such as the following:
  - Sun safety
  - Food safety
  - Sexual behaviors that result in HIV infection, other sexually transmitted diseases, or unintended pregnancy

For More Information   You may interactively complete, download, print, or order copies of the School Health Index on the CDC Web site at www.cdc.gov/HealthyYouth/SHI or request a copy by e-mail at cdcinfo@cdc.gov or by phone at 800-CDC-INFO. When ordering, please specify either the elementary school version or the middle/high school version.

Make It Stick

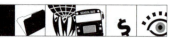

Make It Stick is designed simply to raise awareness by posting reminders about healthy lifestyle behaviors. Sticky notes placed in prominent locations remind people daily of healthy behaviors and good health habits. People often use sticky notes as reminders for daily tasks—why not use them to post health goals?

Goals

- Promote healthy lifestyle behaviors.
- Help people achieve personal health goals.

Description
"I know I should, but . . . ." According to the American Dietetic Association, 40 percent of Americans know about the importance of a healthy diet and what healthy eating behaviors consist of, but they do not practice them. This suggests that many people know what they need to do to stay healthy. But, sometimes life gets in the way. We get busy, we forget or fail to plan ahead, and we may not be successful in achieving healthy lifestyle behaviors. Make It Stick reminds people of the daily things they need to put on their to-do lists to achieve their healthy lifestyle goals. Effective at worksites and in communities and schools, this program creates a buzz and encourages dialogue, which supports the three Vs (see page 27).

People typically need to practice a new health behavior for 21 to 30 days consecutively to adopt it permanently. Therefore, Make It Stick is offered for at least 21 consecutive days. A note may be repeated daily until the behavior is adopted and maintained. However, it is recommended to change notes frequently and not to use the same note for all 21 days. People tend to ignore messages they see over and over again. When a healthy behavior is achieved or adopted permanently, the note or reminder may no longer be needed.

You may launch Make It Stick in an office where colleagues may discuss their personal health goals, share ideas for the achievement of those goals, and support each other. In schools, teachers may encourage students to put notes on their desks or in their day planners. Students may openly discuss their notes or health goals in class and share ideas for accomplishing them. A simple 21-day checklist or calendar may serve as a log for Make It Stick. Participants who complete the calendar for 21 days may turn it in for an incentive such as a raffle ticket.

21 Daily Sticky Note Samples

- Call my doctor to schedule my annual physical.
- Take deep breaths!
- Take a 10-minute walk.
- Look up a healthy recipe for dinner.
- Purchase fruits and vegetables.
- Purchase a lunch box.
- Cut up fruit for tomorrow's lunch or tonight's dessert.
- Make my own healthy lunch to take to work (or school) tomorrow.
- Check out my health insurer's Web site for wellness resources.
- Get at least eight hours of sleep tonight.

- Purchase a good pair of walking or running shoes.
- Enroll in a healthy cooking class.
- Call the doctor about any unusual symptoms I may be ignoring.
- Eat breakfast.
- Recruit an exercise partner.
- Drink eight to ten 8-ounce (237 ml) glasses of water.
- Check my blood pressure.
- Find a healthy snack alternative.
- Eat an apple.
- Avoid foods with trans fats.
- Exercise portion control.

Enhancements

- Have special note pads printed with logos, or purchase apple-shaped sticky note pads for the program.
- Encourage people to sign up, and offer an incentive to anyone who commits to the program for 21 days or more.
- Send out a weekly list of ideas for sticky notes. Ask employees or students to contribute ideas as well.

YMCA's Healthy Family Home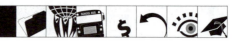

Healthy Family Home is a free, downloadable kit that says, "It's easy (and fun!) to develop healthy habits in three areas." There are three components to Healthy Family Home: Play Every Day, Eat Healthy, and Family Time. The free Healthy Family Home guide provides great ideas to help you get started. This program, created by the YMCA, is about the power of small, sustainable changes for the family. Like many things in life, achieving balance among activities, work, school, and family and friends is challenging, but important. Reach for a variety of tools to support your family, including a variety of physical activities to keep the body and mind interested.

Goals

- Encourage the holistic development of children and youth.
- Improve the health and well-being of children, youth, and families.
- Strengthen family relationships.

Description   "Grown-ups and kids, use this kit to help improve your home environment and jumpstart healthy habits that will lead to a healthier way of living. This kit will support and encourage the whole family in making nurturing, wholesome choices throughout each day. Along with balance and variety, moderation is a key component of a Healthy Family Home. That's why we have fun and tasty sweets as part of our recipe collection. What's life without dessert? But maybe those cookies could be made with less fat, or you could get in the habit of splitting dessert, eating smaller portions, or making healthier substitutions to satisfy your cravings. Choose a variety of foods to keep your taste buds happy."

The goal of this program is to provide families with enough variety in all areas of a Healthy Family Home (Play Every Day, Eat Healthy, and Family Time) that you may pick and choose the tips and activities that make the most sense for your family at any given time and in any given circumstances. This program provides ideas and suggestions, but the real-life changes come from your family's new choices. And remember, it is okay to have a serving of ice cream, it is okay to take a day off from exercise, and it is okay to want some alone time. Healthy Family Home is all about moderate changes here and there that add up to a healthier, happier home environment.

Following are examples from the three components of Healthy Family Home.

Play Every Day   All family members may be role models by following these guidelines:

- Moderate, fun physical activity: Try for at least a total of 60 minutes every day (which may be spread out in 10- to 15-minute intervals), and include outdoor activity whenever possible.
- Vigorous, fun physical activity three days a week: Aim for 20 minutes total on these days, and include outdoor activity whenever possible.
- Bring adults and kids together in physical activities to provide opportunities for connecting and modeling positive behavior.
- Limit screen time to less than two hours per day (i.e., television, video games, computer use). Meals should not be consumed in front of a screen.

Eat Healthy   All family members may be role models by following these guidelines:

- Serve fruits and vegetables at every snack and meal. Offer fresh fruit and vegetable options daily.
- Make water the primary drink option every day. Other options should be non-sugar-sweetened beverages.
- Include a whole grain or protein option with every snack.
- Provide healthy, unsaturated-fat foods at meals and snacks.
- Emphasize balance, variety, and moderation.

Family Time   All family members may be role models by following these guidelines:

- Provide each child with one-to-one time every day.
- Sit down as a family for one meal each day.
- Involve kids in snack and meal preparation and cleanup every day.

Equipment and Supplies

- Healthy Family Home Starter Kit (available free of charge from www.ymca.net/healthyfamilyhome/welcome.html)
- Some of the learning-related activities require simple equipment such as paper, pencils, pedometers, jump ropes, markers, paper products, and food ingredients.

For More Information   For additional information about implementing Healthy Family Home, and to obtain a free Healthy Family Home Starter Kit, visit www.ymca .net/healthyfamilyhome/welcome.html.

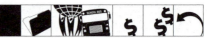
Know Your Numbers is a health screening program designed to inform participants about their personal health status. Screenings may include blood pressure, blood glucose, cholesterol, body mass index (BMI), body weight in relation to height, and body composition or percentage of body fat. A single type of screening or multiple types of screenings may be performed depending on resources, space, and the amount of time participants have available.

Goals

- Screen participants for risk factors for chronic disease (e.g., heart disease, diabetes).
- Assist participants with the interpretation of health screening findings for follow up with personal health care providers.

Description

"If I had any idea my blood pressure was so high, I would have filled the prescription my doctor gave me months ago! I would have gone back for a follow-up visit, but I felt fine!" the employee told the nurse checking blood pressures at a university-based health screening event. As a result of this on-site health screening program, this employee learned about the severity of her blood pressure reading and was advised to go to a nearby phone and call her doctor immediately. If this screening program had not been offered, this woman may have had a serious cardiac event. She explained that her physician had wanted her to return to his office for a blood pressure follow-up a month ago. When asked why she did not return, she stated that she had felt fine and was too busy. On-site screenings may reduce barriers such as lack of time, lack of transportation, lack of health insurance, and high co-payments for office visits that may keep people from seeking routine preventive health care. On-site preventive health care screenings increase participation.

The Know Your Numbers program may be administered in a variety of ways. It may be offered as one stand-alone screening, such as BMI measurements, or as part of a complete suite of biometric screenings, such as BMI, blood pressure, blood glucose, and cholesterol measurements. In-house or qualified nurse contractors may administer the screenings. The price of this program may be kept low by offering only one screening, such as BMI measurements, for which equipment and labor costs are minimal. The program cost may be higher if a complete suite of screenings is offered, especially screenings that require licensed health care professionals. You may arrange for coaches to be available on site to explain results to participants, as well as to offer coaching on how to improve less-than-optimal results. On-site coaching would also warrant additional resources.

When offering this program, keep the following considerations in mind:

- Ensure the security and privacy of personal health data by (1) not saying results out loud, (2) writing results down to give to participants, and (3) positioning tables and waiting lines to ensure the privacy of all participants.
- Ensure that all screening equipment is reserved and that enough staff members are available to minimize waiting lines.
- Set up privacy screens for performing weight measurements.
- Individual biometric or health screenings may be rotated for several consecutive weeks. For example, blood pressure screening on week 1, BMI and body

composition on week 2, cholesterol on week 3, blood glucose on week 4, and so on. Single types of screenings, as opposed to multiple types of screenings, may be well received at sites where employee time is limited, and waiting periods associated with participation in multiple screenings at one event may be a barrier. If multiple screenings are preferred, schedule appointments to avoid long wait times and ensure adequate staff are available.

Enhancements

- Launch an online health risk assessment during Know Your Numbers.
- Have participants enter their screening results directly into their HRQ (see chapter 2) by setting up a computer lab or an additional room with laptops. Have staff available to assist participants with questions.
- If adequate resources and time are available, offer multiple screenings during a single event.
- Contact your organization's health care provider as well as local nonprofit health organizations (e.g., American Heart Association, American Diabetes Association) for assistance.
- Contact local health clubs to request staff assistance.
- Recruit university students enrolled in health majors (e.g., nursing, nutrition, exercise science) for assistance. Know Your Numbers may satisfy clinical or community-based work hour requirements for health majors.

For More Information   Contact your health insurer or your clients' insurer to inquire about assistance with implementing this program.

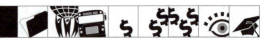

The U.S. Department of Health and Human Services publishes an annual calendar of national health observances that may be used for a wide variety of awareness and educational events in worksite, community, and school settings.

Goal   Increase awareness and knowledge of health topics through national health observances.

Description   An Observe Health program can vary from a poster encouraging people to wear red on National Wear Red Day in February to an annual event. An example of an annual event is the Pink Ribbon Tea held in October (National Breast Cancer Awareness Month), hosted in the beautiful state room at the statehouse by the first lady of Rhode Island, Suzanne Carcieri. China tea cups are placed on round tables with white linens and fresh flowers are wrapped with pink bows. Guests receive a pink ribbon upon entering. The first lady and representatives of the state Breast Cancer Coalition speak on the importance of breast cancer screening and early detection, and the latest advances in treatment. Breast cancer survivors also share their powerful stories of courage and hope.

This type of celebration, which may be conducted at worksites or in communities or schools, is a way to educate others on just one of many health topics with a dedicated national health observance. The cost for this program may vary from low (creating posters or sending out e-mails to raise awareness of the health observance) to high (organizing events that may require speaker fees, food, or entertainment).

Enhancements

- Post an oversized monthly calendar highlighting daily, weekly, or monthly national health observances.
- Take it a step further by offering programs each month in recognition of the specific health topic or observance.
- Contact nonprofit health organizations and ask them to assist with events by sharing health-related materials or offering staff assistance.

For More Information   Download the annual calendar of national health observances at www.healthfinder.gov/nho/default.aspx.

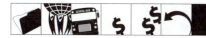

Lactation Support

The U.S. CDC's Healthier Worksite Initiative developed a lactation support toolkit for a worksite Lactation Support program to reduce barriers to breastfeeding among employees who have recently given birth, enabling them to transition back into the workplace while optimizing the benefits their infants receive from being breastfed. Protection, promotion, and support of breastfeeding are critical public health needs. Healthy People 2010, the United States' prevention agenda, set goals for increasing both breastfeeding initiation and duration and decreasing disparities in these rates across all populations in the United States. Increased breastfeeding is also a major program area of the CDC's State-Based Nutrition and Physical Activity Program to Prevent Obesity and Other Chronic Diseases.

Goals

- Increase breastfeeding initiation.
- Increase breastfeeding duration.
- Reduce barriers to breastfeeding among employees who have recently given birth.

Description   According to the CDC, http://www.cdc.gov/breastfeeding/pdf/breastfeeding_interventions.pdf mothers are the fastest-growing segment of the U.S. labor force. Approximately 70 percent of employed mothers with children younger than three years work full-time. One-third of these mothers return to work within three months after birth, and two-thirds return within six months. Working outside the home is related to a shorter duration of breastfeeding, and intentions to work full-time are significantly associated with lower rates of breastfeeding initiation and shorter duration. Given the substantial presence of mothers in the workforce, there is a strong need to establish lactation support in the workplace. Barriers identified in the workplace include a lack of flexibility for milk expression in the work schedule, lack of accommodations to pump or store breast milk, concerns about support from employers and colleagues, and real or perceived low milk supply.

The cost of implementing this program varies from low to medium. An organization may simply implement a lactation support policy at no cost, offer lactation support services, or establish a designated lactation room.

Lactation Support Toolkit   The CDC Lactation Support toolkit is available free of cost online at www.cdc.gov/nccdphp/dnpa/hwi/toolkits/lactation/. It provides an example of how to create a comprehensive lactation, or breastfeeding, support program for nursing mothers at the worksite. The term *lactation support program* is intended to signify a program that provides lactating employees with educational and environmental support of their breastfeeding goals. The toolkit is designed to help employers set up a program for employees to be able to pump and store their breast milk at work, to take home to their infants at the end of the workday.

Kathleen Cullinen, PhD, RD, LDN, former director of the Rhode Island Obesity Prevention and Control Program, states, "This is a comprehensive toolkit that provides states with the resources to institute policy and environmental supports for increasing breastfeeding, a national strategy for reducing childhood obesity and related chronic diseases."

>> continued

Toolkit Components The toolkit describes how federal and nonfederal workplaces may plan and implement a comprehensive Lactation Support program and evaluate its success. Three topics are covered in the toolkit: lactation-supportive policies, lactation support services (such as breast pumps or breastfeeding classes and support groups), and creating a physical environment that supports lactation. The toolkit describes the following project phases:

- Assessing need and interest
- Planning
- Implementing
- Maintaining
- Evaluating

Enhancements

- Provide educational materials to employers about how supporting their employees who breastfeed benefits employers.
- Establish a model Lactation Support program for all state employees.
- Promote legislation to support worksite lactation programs through mandates or incentives.
- Create worksite recognition programs to honor employers who support their breastfeeding employees.

For More Information Visit www.cdc.gov/nccdphp/dnpa/hwi/toolkits/lactation/.

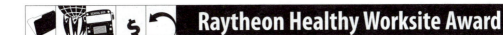

To acknowledge and reward its locations that are actively engaged in supporting and improving the health of employees, Raytheon instituted the Raytheon Healthy Worksite Award program. This award program encourages site implementation of Raytheon wellness initiatives, promotes and demonstrates site leadership support for a culture of health and well-being, and drives employee participation.

Goals

- Improve the culture of health and well-being at various sites.
- Strengthen program infrastructure.
- Improve program participation and engagement.

Description   Competitive award and recognition programs may be powerful motivators to drive engagement and positive program outcomes. Consider adding an award and recognition program to your wellness initiative, particularly if you work for a large organization with various departments or divisions, or for an organization with multiple or satellite locations. If you don't have funding for financial incentives, awards and recognition are a strategy for motivating people. An award program that publicly recognizes successful program participation and health outcomes may also help build a strong culture of wellness within any organization or community. An award program must be well thought out, clearly defined, and well communicated. It must provide equal opportunity for all participants.

Criteria for the Raytheon Healthy Worksite Award program serve as a great model for an award program. Consider focus areas specific to your organization's wellness goals and objectives, and develop customized criteria to achieve them. Raytheon has multiple sites and locations, and the award criteria they have developed identify sites with the most outstanding wellness programs. You can modify the following criteria of the Raytheon Healthy Worksite Award program to fit your organization's needs:

- Leadership support
- Wellness team engagement and effectiveness
- Wellness program operating plan and budget
- Wellness programs that address general health and well-being, weight management, physical activity, nutrition, tobacco use, stress management, and ergonomic injury prevention
- Workplace environment and policies (e.g., healthy food choices, tobacco policy enforcement, fitness resources)
- Site participation in the health risk assessment or questionnaire (HRQ)
- Participation metrics for various programs

Equipment

- Award program description and application
- Team to review applications
- Plaques or other tangible awards to give to qualifying sites

Enhancement   Progressively increase the requirements for each of the award levels.

For More Information   Visit www.raytheon.com/responsibility/stewardship/wellness/index.html.

Wellness Impact Scorecard

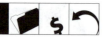

The National Business Group on Health offers the Wellness Impact Scorecard ("Scorecard"), an online tool to help employers evaluate the impact of their health improvement programs on their workforce's overall health. The Scorecard is unique in that it advances wellness program evaluation from counting health risks to measuring healthy behaviors in order to improve the health status of employees.

Goals

- Identify appropriate metrics to evaluate the impact of wellness programs.
- Track and report progress on key process and outcome measures.
- Recommend new components of wellness programs or performance improvement.
- Benchmark wellness programs with peer companies over time (i.e., longitudinal program evaluation).

Description   In consultation with leading researchers in wellness and worksite health promotion, the National Business Group on Health developed an online Wellness Impact Scorecard that allows companies to assess and improve their wellness programs while comparing them with those of other organizations and proven best practices. The program is free for members. Specifically, employers need to be asking the following:

- Are these at-risk groups improving their health behaviors?
- Are healthy behaviors already in place being maintained?
- Is the employee population moving toward overall better health status?

For More Information   To join the National Business Group on Health and obtain a copy of the Scorecard, contact benchmarking@businessgrouphealth.org, or visit www.businessgrouphealth.org/scorecard.

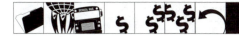
Alfa Laval partnered with Preventure, a full-service wellness company, to design an incentive program to engage more employees in their comprehensive employee health and wellness program, ALwell Incentives. Alfa Laval believes that the success of the company depends on its employees. With this in mind, it has developed an employee wellness program whose mission is to "promote and support employee welfare by providing opportunities to enhance awareness, encourage positive lifestyle changes, and improve the quality of life resulting in a healthier and more productive workforce." ALwell Incentives helps make wellness programs exciting for employees and results in higher participation rates. The cost for this program ranges from $40 to $150 per eligible participant per year. This incentive concept may be applied to programs in community or school settings as well.

Goals

- Engage employees to participate in a health and wellness program.
- Increase the percentage of participants who receive preventive exams.
- Reduce the percentage of employees at risk for unhealthy behaviors.

Description   Employee engagement in the ALwell Incentives program is ensured through a strategic incentive strategy. Two categories of employee incentives are provided—Healthy Habits and Wellness Credits. Together, they increase employee interest in wellness programs and motivate employees to live healthier lifestyles. The credits, based on points, are accumulated over a one-year period. Points are tracked by Preventure using an online tracking system. Predetermined activities generate points, such as completing a health risk assessment or questionnaire (HRQ), participating in a community road race, completing a smoking cessation program, or completing preventive screenings.

Healthy Habits   Healthy Habits is a credit-based incentive program that encourages participation in the components of a wellness program. Wellness components might be health risk assessments or questionnaires (HRQs), health or biometric screenings, wellness workshops, or walking challenges. Healthy Habits rewards employees and their spouses who already make good wellness choices, and motivates those who are just getting started. Because Healthy Habits incentives are about efforts and not results, everyone has an opportunity to earn credits. Employees earn points for each wellness activity they complete (there are about 50 options) and earn the following wellness credits based on their total points:

- First Step = $50; 8 activities completed by employee or spouse
- Pacing Yourself = $100; 15 activities completed by employee or spouse
- Full Stride = $150; 22 activities completed by employee or spouse

Wellness Credits   ALwell Incentives provides the opportunity to earn wellness credits for completing a wellness assessment, joining a health club, working out at a health club, or participating in the Healthy Habits incentive program. Credits earned may be used during open enrollment to reduce benefit costs, deposited into the employee's 401k account, or received as taxable income. Various amounts or credits are assigned

>> continued

to key activities identified by the organization as a health priority or health risk–based decision-making process.

Employees are empowered with many resources to improve their knowledge, lifestyles, and overall health, including the following:

- Health assessment
- Biometric screenings
- ALwell Web portal
- Lifestyle coaching
- Weight management program
- Tobacco cessation program
- Employee assistance program
- International fitness club network

- Incentives for enrolling in or using a health club
- Lunch and Learn seminars
- Flu shots
- LunchWell program
- Health awareness newsletters
- Wellness challenges
- Wellness team

Enhancement   All programs are updated annually to ensure that they continue to strategically support wellness program goals, keep employees interested and engaged, and improve employee and family health.

For More Information   Visit www.preventure.com or contact Preventure at 888-321-4326. Additional information on health management incentive programs may also be obtained from insurance providers, health and wellness consultants, and other independent vendors.

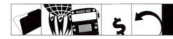

A New Look at Why I Smoke and How to Quit

For most people, smoking is more than a habit; thus, it takes a broad understanding of the effects of nicotine to support those motivated to quit. To help those seeking to quit, the Know Your Health: A New Look at Why I Smoke and How to Quit program provides comprehensive education about smoking. Topics discussed in this free program include current prevalence statistics, physiological and social effects, federal and state policies, health consequences, and steps and tools that are available to help people quit.

Goals

- Increase awareness of the health problems caused by smoking cigarettes.
- Educate participants on the benefits of quitting and maintaining a smoke-free life.
- Identify and understand motivators for smoking.
- Educate participants on the options for quitting smoking.
- Enable participants to choose the right individualized plan to quit and stay quit with physician or other health care provider support.

Description   Know Your Health is a health literate education program that focuses on prevention and wellness. The smoking cessation module, A New Look at Why I Smoke and How to Quit, contains the following materials:

- *Smoking Cessation and More Than a Habit* CD-ROM, and facilitator and promotional materials, including facilitator guides, facilitator PowerPoint presentations, and promotional posters
- My Health Account: A New Look at Why I Smoke and How to Quit
- Completion certificates for host organization and participants

By using Know Your Health: A New Look at Why I Smoke and How to Quit, sponsored by Pfizer Inc., you may reach a broad audience of smokers and help them quit. The program consists of components that may be used together or individually and includes facilitator guides, facilitator PowerPoint presentations, an educational brochure, promotional posters, and completion certificates. The facilitator guides and CD-ROM contain the following two PowerPoint presentations (with accompanying lecture notes):

1. **Professional presentation:** To assist hospitals, health systems, payer groups, employers, physicians, and policy makers with formulating a plan to support quitters.
2. **Consumer presentation:** To educate the general public (e.g., employees and patients). The main target audience for the program is smokers who are motivated to quit.

>> continued

A pocket-sized educational brochure helps smokers become aware of the health problems caused by smoking. The brochure provides tools to help smokers quit.

The promotional posters are designed to draw an audience to an educational program (using the consumer or professional PowerPoint presentations included on the CD-ROM). The posters are also included on the CD-ROM. The posters may be customized with the date, time, and location of the program, then printed and displayed by the host of the program.

For More Information   To receive items needed for Know Your Health: A New Look at Why I Smoke and How to Quit, contact your local Pfizer director of employers, account manager, or medical outcomes specialist, or contact the Pfizer corporate office at 212-733-2323.

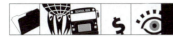

My Pledge

My Pledge is an awareness program that may be offered in a variety of settings at minimal to no cost. In this program, people in a group setting publicly declare to their peers their commitment to personal health by pledging to engage in certain positive health behaviors. Publicly pledging one's commitment to engage in positive health behaviors is a very effective health promotion strategy.

Goals

- Increase awareness of healthy lifestyle behaviors.
- Increase commitment to and responsibility for personal health.
- Improve health behaviors.

Description   Simply put, My Pledge is a an awareness program that encourages members of an organization or group to visibly post their commitment to personal health improvement as a pledge on a large bulletin board displayed in a visible, central location for all to see (see the three Vs in chapter 2). Setting up this program simply requires written or verbal requests of potential participants to post their pledges on the bulletin board. Participants will need index cards to write their pledges on, along with pushpins to post them. If your bulletin board cannot accommodate an excessive number of pledges or index cards, you may remove them daily, every other day, or weekly and store them in an index card box for future posting or as a follow-up at the end of the program. Alternatively, pledges may be posted for one month. Don't let pledges get stale. Consider rotating older pledges to the bottom of the bulletin board and posting more current pledges at the top to keep messaging fresh.

At the top of the bulletin board post or write MY PLEDGE. Provide instructions on or near the bulletin board for writing pledges on index cards, signing them, dating them, and posting them on the bulletin board. Post sample pledges on or near the bulletin board.

Additional tips on implementing My Pledge include the following:

- Ask senior leaders within your worksite, community, or school to demonstrate senior-leader support by posting their pledges. This sets an example and gets the process started.

- Ask one person to post a pledge, and then ask that person to ask someone else to post a pledge, and so on.

- Send an e-mail to all employees, clients, or students inviting all to write and sign their pledges on the bulletin board demonstrating their commitment to a personal, positive health behavior change.

- The bulletin board or flip chart may be changed weekly (or more frequently if necessary if there are many pledges) to provide more ideas and encourage people to keep adding to their personal pledges. You can post full bulletin boards or flip chart sheets in cafeterias, hallways, or other highly visible, high-traffic areas, or rotate pledge cards on the bulletin board and store those removed for later use as described earlier.

>> continued

My Pledge ideas include the following:

- I pledge to park my car farther away from my destination.
- I pledge to take stairs instead of elevators.
- I pledge to eat at least five servings of fruits and vegetables per day.
- I pledge to walk more throughout the course of my day.
- I pledge to exercise three times this week.
- I pledge to join an exercise class.
- I pledge to go for my annual physical exam.
- I pledge to have my mammogram this month.

Enhancements

- My Pledge may supplement any health campaign.
- People can sign one-page pledge sheets pertaining to a specific health behavior change posted on office or classroom doors, in cafeterias, hallways, or other highly visible, high-traffic areas.

For More Information

- Visit www.projectappleseed.org/pledgefitnessnutrition.html to see an example of an online pledge form.
- Visit *stickK* (www.stickk.com/), an online social networking site that allows you to put a "contract out on yourself" by publicly committing to your health and wellness goals.

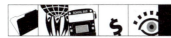

Virtual Reminders

Virtual Reminders is an e-mail messaging program designed by the wellness ambassador for Hewitt's virtual associates. Hewitt's virtual associates, or those working from remote locations across North America, stay connected with one another through brief e-mail messages that promote healthy lifestyle behaviors. Members of the team alternate responsibility for crafting and e-mailing an evidence-based health prompt to the group each day for 30 days. With 35 virtual associates, each associate is required to contribute only one healthy lifestyle message during a 30-day time frame.

Goals
- Promote healthy lifestyle behaviors.
- Engage employees in wellness.
- Promote teamwork.

Description   Megan Ruane, a consultant for Hewitt Associates and wellness ambassador for Hewitt's virtual associates in North America, designed Virtual Reminders as a strategy to virtually engage her team in the Hewitt wellness initiative Choose Health. Choose Health is a comprehensive wellness initiative with open enrollment that includes a health risk questionnaire (HRQ), incentives, health coaching, wellness programming, measurement, and evaluation. Virtual Reminders was developed as a response to the challenge of keeping Hewitt's virtual associates, dispersed and working remotely across North America, engaged in Choose Health. It is a simple, very low-cost, daily e-mail reminder program that has proven to be highly effective at involving all team members in health promotion and wellness. On his or her assigned day, each team member e-mails a health-related tip, motivational quote, personal anecdote, healthy recipe, or daily health challenge to all team members.

Here are some sample daily Virtual Reminders:

- Eat three servings of fruit.
- Do 25 sit-ups before bed.
- Drink 64 ounces (2 l) of water in a day.
- Attached is my favorite recipe for a fruit smoothie. Try this simple and tasty recipe this week!
- I have days when I just don't want to work out, for whatever reason. However, I was able to find a way to continue my commitment to wellness by recently participating in a charity run, which was very inspirational. I encourage all of you to find a wellness or fitness activity that motivates and challenges you!
- Add high-fiber ingredients to your food or recipes to help you feel fuller longer.
- I always keep canned chickpeas in the house. They are a great, mild-tasting addition to soups, sauces, and salads!
- Go for a 30-minute walk after dinner tonight.

Enhancements
- Send invitations to organizational members to join Virtual Reminders.
- Form groups of participants and assign a day of the week or month (depending on the number of participants) to each participant.
- Wellness champions may organize Virtual Reminders at their worksite, in their community, or at their school.

Vitality

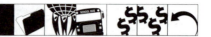

For more than 70 years, Ottawa Dental Laboratory has taken great pride in offering its 120 employees the best health care benefits available. However, four years ago, rising health care costs and a string of double-digit premium increases reached unsustainable levels. The management team was committed to finding a solution. Ottawa Dental adopted a Web- and incentive-based health improvement program, provided by Vitality, a health enhancement solution company. This program uses a personalized approach and rewards members for engaging in behaviors that lower their health risks and help them achieve measurable clinical improvements in health indicators such as blood pressure, blood glucose, and cholesterol. The cost is approximately $3 per person per month. Price may vary depending on the services and incentives offered.

Goals

- Improve employee health and fitness.
- Reduce health care costs.
- Increase participation in wellness activities.

Description   Vitality addresses clinically documented drivers of health risk and provides appropriate incentives across the entire population, regardless of health status, age, and physical ability. It helps to keep Ottawa Dental's members out of the health care system and delays the progression of disease for those at most risk. When Ottawa began working with Vitality in 2004, employees were offered incentives to complete a health risk assessment and participate in preventive screenings. Many potentially serious problems were discovered during this process, including two cases of serious heart problems that the people did not know they had. Each employee received suggestions for risk-reducing activities, such as exercise, nutrition education, and smoking cessation, and were motivated by incentives, or bucks (redeemable for personalized rewards), to take action. For example, an employee who completes a health risk assessment is awarded 1,000 bucks. Bucks are awarded for everything from completing the initial health risk assessment to working out and completing an annual physical. Employees are also awarded for achieving their health goals. Bucks may be redeemed for a variety of rewards from movie tickets to more expensive items such as flat screen televisions.

Ottawa Dental recognized that the main challenge with most wellness programs is that employees who need them most do not participate. As such, management took into consideration the following critical factors when identifying and developing the program:

- **Depends on management involvement and support.** Ottawa's president and other senior staff members demonstrate ongoing support of the program and work out with employees at a gym that is part of the integrated program.
- **Offers proper and nondiscriminatory incentives.** The program has four participation levels. The more people accomplish, the more rewards they earn. In addition, employees earn bucks, redeemable for a variety of rewards, so they may choose rewards most appealing to them. Employees, regardless of their initial state of health, are given equal opportunity to earn rewards.

- **Personalized approach is designed to stretch across the spectrum of health.** Vitality provides a personalized approach for every employee. For example, the focus for healthy people may be promoting physical activity, whereas for those at risk, the focus may be lowering cholesterol or enrolling in a disease management program.

- **Addresses all major risk factors.** Vitality is designed to address clinically documented drivers of health risk.

- **Is inspirational, fun, and easy to use.** Vitality appeals to employees at all health levels, and the variety of incentives makes it engaging.

This program may be offered at worksites and in communities and schools by partnering with the vendor or by designing a similar program internally in which wellness bucks may be assigned to certain programs and offerings.

Equipment   Vitality requires employee access to the Internet.

For More Information   Visit www.vitality.com/. Information on similar incentive-based health improvement programs may also be obtained from insurance providers, health and wellness consultants, and other independent vendors.

Healthy Book Club

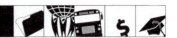

Healthy Book Club is an informative group education program. It provides a forum for questions and discussions of solutions to barriers to positive behavior change, offers group social support, and may provide proper demonstrations of the techniques and recommendations outlined in the books reviewed. Healthy Book Club also provides accountability; participants read material prior to group meetings, which, in itself, may attract new participants to other wellness programs.

Goals

- Increase knowledge of health and wellness topics.
- Provide social support through weekly group meetings.

Description

Healthy Book Club may be held at worksites during lunch or after work; in community settings such as hospitals, health clubs, senior centers, and recreation centers; or in school or after-school settings for children and parents. Regularly scheduled meetings provide the opportunity to gather and discuss a book or other reading related to health and wellness. Healthy snacks are also provided. The facilitator, a personal trainer or health educator, assigns homework, presents the content of that week's assignment for group discussion, answers questions, and provides input and feedback on the material. Participants share their successes regarding the healthy lifestyle practices covered, barriers they experienced, and how they overcame them. When the club is discussing books on exercise, the group practices the exercises together and the facilitator corrects form or demonstrates modifications. Suggested books available at www.humankinetics.com/ include the following:

- *Fit in 5: 5, 10 & 30 Minute Workouts for a Leaner, Stronger Body* by Greg Whyte
- *Nancy Clark's Sports Nutrition Guidebook, Fourth Edition,* by Nancy Clark
- *Running Well* by Sam Murphy and Sarah Connors
- *Strength Ball Training, Second Edition,* by Lorne Goldenberg and Peter Twist
- *Beth Shaw's YogaFit, Second Edition,* by Beth Shaw

Enhancements

- Prepare a suggested reading list and have members vote on book selections and reading order.
- Provide incentives for completing assignments such as a free book to be covered in the next Healthy Book Club meeting.
- Invite family members to participate.
- Augment the content of books (e.g., the facilitator may add a weekly meditation component to a stress management book review).
- As a marketing strategy for health clubs or other organizations, open up Healthy Book Club to nonmembers.

A component of the state of Delaware's comprehensive wellness program, DelaWELL University is a worksite health education program that encompasses the following four health topics: physical activity, weight management, stress management, and nutrition. It may be implemented at worksites and in community-based organizations, as well as schools.

Goals

- Increase physical activity.
- Achieve and maintain a healthy body weight.
- Reduce stress.
- Improve nutrition.

Description

In 2007–2008, health risk assessment or questionnaire (HRQ) results from the state of Delaware's comprehensive wellness program, DelaWELL, indicated that lack of physical activity, overweight and obesity, stress, and poor nutrition were among the most prevalent risk factors for chronic disease within the employee population. Determined to target and positively influence these high-risk areas, in 2008 the state of Delaware's DelaWELL program launched its comprehensive health education program DelaWELL University. The program encourages employees to attend a series of the following four health seminars: (1) The Active Workday, (2) Managing Your Weight, (3) Stress and Your Workday, and (4) Eating for Performance and Health. This program provides an overall sense of academic achievement; the ability to graduate to a better level of health; and attractive, low-cost incentives or giveaways such as pedometers, T-shirts, mugs, beach towels, and lunch tote bags.

The cost of this program may be minimal, with the exception of occasionally reserving state vehicles for transportation to and from seminars. When possible, diplomas may be printed in-house using regular white paper and colored ink. Diploma distribution may be done through state interoffice mail at no cost. Low-cost incentives or giveaways may be purchased or donated.

Each of the four one-hour health seminars are offered over a period of two months at 24 state and school district locations, either during lunchtime or after school, to accommodate employees' varying work schedules. Multiple communication modalities including e-mails, posters, flyers, and a Web site are used to actively promote the program. Employees may register online for the seminar of their choice and receive an automated confirmation e-mail. One week prior to each seminar, an e-mail reminder notice is sent to all registrants. Seminars are taught by a member of the statewide wellness office and include a PowerPoint presentation, educational handouts, and an exit survey. Employees who attend one session in each of the four health seminar topics receive a DelaWELL University diploma signed by the governor (which demonstrates senior-level support) to commend their outstanding dedication and commitment to learning about and improving their personal health and well-being. Participants also have the opportunity to win a personalized nutritional analysis by a registered dietitian, and giveaway items at each seminar.

>> continued

Supplies

- An online registration mechanism with data collecting and reporting capabilities. (A sample online registration form is available at https://delaware.online.staywell.com/includes/login/index.aspx.) If computer programming support is available, a back-end data collection application may be developed.

- A paper-based registration may be used with manual data collection (see the sample form on page 167). A simple Microsoft Excel spreadsheet may be manually set up to track registration information and program attendance.

- Adequate classroom space with enough tables and chairs to accommodate participants.

- If necessary, transportation to and from seminar locations.

- Audiovisual equipment, including a laptop or computer, projector, and if necessary, a microphone with an attached speaker system for larger areas.

- A registered dietitian to donate personalized nutritional analyses for winners of four random drawings.

Enhancements

- Offer additional health seminar topics such as self-care, managing back pain, high blood pressure, high blood cholesterol, and smoking cessation.

- Offer late afternoon or evening seminars.

- Provide other incentives such as free trial memberships to local fitness centers or cooking classes.

- Conduct a follow-up survey of participants to measure behavior change and program satisfaction.

For More Information   Visit http://delawell.delaware.gov/.

Seminar Registration Form

{Include program logo here, if available}

Thank you for your interest in our program. Please fill out this form in its entirety and e-mail or fax a completed copy to [insert the appropriate contact's name and number] to register.

Have questions regarding this form? Please contact [insert the appropriate contact's name and number].

Seminar title: _____

Seminar date: _____

Seminar location: _____

First name: _____

Last name: _____

Work telephone: _____

Work e-mail address: _____

Department/division/unit: _____

Work address: _____

City: _____

State: _____

Zip code: _____

Interoffice mail code: _____

❑   Please check the box if you are interested in receiving information on future wellness programs.

From A. Ludovici-Connolly, 2010, *Winning health promotion strategies* (Champaign, IL: Human Kinetics).

Screen Savers

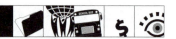

Screen Savers is a health awareness program to increase healthy lifestyle behaviors throughout the work- or school day.

Goal

Improve lifestyle behaviors and health habits.

Description

The phrase *Stop, Stretch, and Breathe* moves across the computer screen. A screen saver (which supports the three Vs in chapter 2) reminds Sharon, a budget analyst working in a stressful state budget office, to take a few minutes every few hours to stop, stretch, and breathe to improve her breathing, reduce her mental and physical tension, and reduce her stress level. Putting a visual reminder on the computer screen at her desk prompts Sharon to perform a healthy behavior in the midst of a narrow focus on her primary task at hand—budget development and review. Sometimes at work or school, we may get so focused on our work, that we disregard any thoughts of incorporating healthy lifestyle behaviors into our daily schedules. Given that the average workweek has increased to 50 hours, it becomes even more important to integrate good health habits into our daily lives.

Here are some sample screen savers:

- Take a 10-minute walk.
- Look up a healthy recipe for dinner.
- Get at least eight hours of sleep tonight.
- Eat breakfast.
- Drink eight to ten 8-ounce (237 ml) glasses of water today.
- Check my blood pressure.
- Eat an apple.

Enhancements

- Distribute a list of screen savers. Ask participants to select one per month to display on their computers.
- As a school project, ask students to create their own screen savers to display on their computers each week or month.
- Create screen savers of photos of employees or students engaging in healthy lifestyle behaviors.

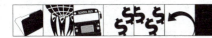

TrestleTree Health Coaching

Health coaching in its purest form is about helping people individually change unhealthy behaviors. Health coaching in its most rigorous form is helping less motivated or unmotivated people individually change unhealthy behaviors. Health coaching is both an art and a science. The science addresses leveraging evidence-based guidelines to direct each participant's goals. The art involves health coaches with dynamic influencing skills helping people experience health behavior changes that may be measured and sustained, which will directly decrease health care costs and provide a positive return on investment (ROI).

The average annual cost of the TrestleTree Health Coaching program varies between $150 and $300 per participant.

Goals

- Enrollment: Increase the percentage of eligible at-risk people who join to more than 50 percent.
- Participation: Increase the percentage of participants who actively work with a coach to more than 80 percent.
- Changed health behaviors: Increase the percentage of participants who change their behaviors to more than 50 percent.
- ROI: Achieve savings and ROI in a timely manner (less than a year and a half).

Description   TrestleTree Health Coaching programs are not a preset number of interventions, but allow participants to participate long enough to measurably change their poor health behaviors. TrestleTree coaches are trained to establish a relationship of trust with each participant so that they will be more effective at supporting positive behavior change. The impact on the health of participants from a trucking company over eight years showed an average weight loss of 19 pounds (8.6 kg), an increase in regular exercise from 25 to 62 percent, and a tobacco cessation rate of 52 percent. Ninety-three percent of the participants reported reduced stress, and average laboratory test results shifted from above normal ranges to within normal ranges.

Enhancement   TrestleTree has partnerships with online coaching programs, biometric screening companies, and at-home monitoring companies that provide additional depth to the core TrestleTree Health Coaching programs. Offering a premium differential as an incentive to participate in Your Health Story (a live telephonic health assessment) has been successful at achieving greater than 95 percent participation.

For More Information   Visit www.trestletree.com or call 866-523-8185. Information on similar health coaching programs may also be obtained from insurance providers, health and wellness consultants, and other independent vendors.

Andreasen AR. (1995). *Marketing social change: changing behavior to promote health, social development, and the environment.* San Francisco, CA: Jossey-Bass.

Bandura A. (1994). "Self-efficacy". In V. S. Ramachaudran (Ed.), *Encyclopedia of human behavior* (Vol. 4, pp. 71-81). New York: Academic Press. Reprinted in H. Friedman [Ed.], *Encyclopedia of mental health,* San Diego: Academic Press, 1998.

Bandura A. (1997). *Self efficacy: The exercise of control.* New York, NY: W.H. Freeman and Company.

Chenoweth D. (2007). *Worksite health promotion.* Champaign, IL: Human Kinetics.

Christakis NA, Fowler JH. (2007). The spread of obesity in a large social network over 32 years. *New England Journal of Medicine*, 357(4): 370-379.

Collins J. (2001). *Good to great.* New York, NY: HarperCollins.

Collins JJ, Porras. (1977). *Built to last: Successful habits of visionary companies.* New York, NY: HarperCollins.

Cox C. (2003). *ACSM's worksite health promotion manual.* Champaign, IL: Human Kinetics.

Cyzman D, Wierenga J, Sielawa J. (2009). A community response to the food environment. *Health Promot Pract.* Apr;10(2 Suppl):146S-155S. PubMed PMID: 19454761.

Edington D. (2009). *Zero trends.* Health Management Research Center. Ann Arbor, Michigan: University of Michigan.

Glicksman AS, Meyer A, DiPiero M, Cullinen K. (in press). Breast health for seniors: Increasing mammography use among older women in Rhode Island. *Journal of Cancer Education.*

Goetzel R, Guindon A, Turshen IJ, Ozminkowski R. (2001). Health and productivity management: Establishing key performance measures, benchmarks, and best practices. *Journal of Occupational and Environmental Medicine* 43:10-17.

Goetzel RZ, Anderson DR, Whitmer RW, Ozminkowski RJ, Dunn RL, Wasserman J. (1998). Health Enhancement Research Organization (HERO) Research Committee. The relationship between modifiable health risks and health care expenditures. An analysis of the multi-employer HERO health risk and cost database. *Journal of Occupational & Environmental Medicine* 40(10):843-54.

Kerr NA, Yore MM, Ham SA, Dietz WH. (2004). Increasing stair use in a worksite through environmental changes. *American Journal of Health Promotion* 18(4): 312-315.

Meyers DG, Neuberger JS, He J. (2009). Cardiovascular effect of bans on smoking in public places: A systematic review and meta-analysis. *Journal of the American College of Cardiology* 54 (14): 1249-1255.

Murray CJL, Lopez AD, eds. (1996). *The global burden of disease and injury series, volume 1: A comprehensive assessment of mortality and disability from diseases, injuries, and risk factors in 1990 and projected to 2020.* Cambridge, MA: Published by the Harvard School of Public Health on behalf of the World Health Organization and the World Bank, Harvard University Press.

Prochaska JJ, Nigg CR, Spring B, Velicer WF, Prochaska JO. (2009). The benefits and challenges of multiple health behavior change in research and in practice. *Preventive Medicine*, Dec 4.

Prochaska JO, Norcross JC, DiClemente C. (2006). *Changing for good.* New York, NY: HarperCollins.

Prochaska JO, Velicer WF, Rossi JS, Goldstein MG, Marcus BH, Rakowski W, Fiore C, Harlow LL, Redding CA, Rosenbloom D. (1994). Stages of change and decisional balance for 12 problem behaviors. *Journal of Health Psychology*, Jan;13(1): 39-46.

Pronk N. (2009). *ACSM's worksite health handbook.* 2nd ed. Champaign, IL: Human Kinetics.

Sallis JF, Hovell MF. (1990). Determinants of exercise behavior. *Exercise and Sport Sciences Reviews*, Jan 18(1): 307-330.

Sallis JF, Hovell MF, Hofstetter CR, Barrington E. (1992). Explanation of vigorous physical activity during two years using social learning variables. *Social Science & Medicine*, Jan;34(1): 25-32.

Schmidt WD, Biwer CJ, Kalscheuer LK. (2001). Effects of long versus short bout exercise on fitness and weight loss in overweight females. *Journal of the American College of Nutrition*, 20 (5): 494-501.

Seaverson EL, Grossmeier J, Miller TM, Anderson D. (2009). The Role of Incentive Design, Incentive Value, Communications Strategy, and Worksite Culture on Health Risk Assessment Participation. *American Journal of Health Promotion*: Vol. 23, No. 5, pp. 343-352.

Smedley BD, Syme SL, eds., (2000). A social environmental approach to health and health interventions. In: *Promoting Health: Intervention Strategies from Social and Behavioral Research*. Washington, D.C.: National Academy Press.

Taitel MS, Haufle V, Heck D, Loeppke R, Fetterolf D. (2008). Incentives and other factors associated with employee participation in health risk assessments. *Journal of Occupational and Environmental Medicine*. Aug;50(8): 863-72.

Ulmer DD. (1984). Societal influences on health and life-styles, in Personal Health Maintenance [Special Issue]. *West J Med,* 1984 Dec; 141: 793-798.

Watanabe N, Stewart R, Jenkins R, Bhugra DK, Furukawa TA. (2008). The epidemiology of chronic fatigue, physical illness, and symptoms of common mental disorders: a cross-sectional survey from the second British national survey of psychiatric morbidity. *Journal of Psychosomatic Research*, 2008 Apr;64(4): 357-62.

World Health Organization. *The world health report 2008. Primary care—now more than ever.* http:www.who.int/whr/2008/en/index.html. Accessed January 6, 2010.

Note: The italicized *f* following page numbers refers to the figure on that page, respectively.

10-10-10 88-89
15 for 15 124

A

ABC for Fitness 12, 90
absenteeism 28, 74
ACSM's Worksite Health Promotion Manual (Cox) 18, 32, 73
Active Living 52
Active Living Every Day 84-85
advertising. *See* social marketing
advisory boards 19, 26
advocacy 10
AEI programming 18, 36, 72
alcohol consumption 75
Alere 66
All You Can Eat 119-120
alternative therapies 10
ALwell Incentives 155-156
American College of Sports Medicine 50
American Heart Association 39
American Idol 37
American Lung Association 38
Americans with Disabilities Act (ADA) 32, 40
An Apple a Day 114
Andreasen, A. 49
Arkansas 6
aromatherapy 48
awareness programs 18, 36, 38

B

Bandura, Albert 62, 63
barriers
   cultural 65
   discretionary time 8
   language 65
   perceived 8
   to physical activity participation 64
   program related 64, 65
   technology 32, 65
behavior change. *See also* incentives
   barriers to 64-65
   engagement for 72
   learning 62
   long-term 65
   maintenance of 38
   pros of 65
   readiness 31, 36, 60

social-ecological model 76*f*
and societal influences 63-64
stages of 60
theories of 59-60
voluntary 50
behaviors
   consumer 49
   high-risk 75
   and interpretation of physiological cues 63
   modeling 63
   preventing relapse 38
   prompting 38
   reminders 38
benchmarks 17, 18, 79
best practices 17, 18
beverages
   in schools 77
   in vending machines 77
beverage samples 48
bike paths 78
biometric screenings 10, 28, 33
blood glucose 33
blood pressure 33
Blue Cross Blue Shield of Rhode Island 7
body mass index 33
Breast Health for Seniors 134
Brown University 45
budgeting 36, 39, 58
Built to Last (Collins and Porras) 74
bulletin boards 48, 78
business sector 6
business strategy 17

C

cafeterias 77
Carcieri, Donald L., Governor 7, 19
Carcieri, Suzanne, First Lady of RI 7, 20, 24
CDCynergy 50
Centers for Disease Control and Prevention (CDC) 50, 52, 76, 79
Chaet, Mike 57
children. *See also* schools

engaging parents 11, 12
   obesity 11
cholesterol 33, 65
Choose Well-Live Well 54
chronic disease 4, 51, 52, 59
cigarette tax 77
clock building 74
Club Med 44, 45
Collins, J. 22, 72, 74
Colossal Colon 138-139
communication. *See also* wellness promotion
   brochures 12, 38, 39, 48, 53
   delivery methods 55, 78
   newsletters 39, 54
   and organizational culture 27
   organization-wide 17
   reminder systems 38
   skills 23
   through Web sites 23
   via e-mail 20, 23, 38, 55
   of vision 73
   visual 27, 31, 38
communities
   environmental approach 78
   policies 77
   programs 9-10
   resources in 10
community assessments 79
Community College of Rhode Island (CCRI) 46
Community Cookbook 115
community directory 5
community planning 6
comprehensive initiatives 18
computers
   access to 32
   for online assessments 32
   proficiency barrier 32, 65
   workstations 28, 52
consciousness raising 61
consultants 6. *See also* wellness professionals
cooking demonstrations 48
Cooper Institute 52
cost savings 18, 74
counter-conditioning 62
Cox, C. 18, 32, 73

Cryer, Michael, Dr. 37
cultural sensitivity 22, 52

D

dance programs 9, 104
data 18, 71
　baseline 28
　collecting 17, 74, 75
　demographic 51, 52
　evaluating 34, 75
　relevance 75
　self-reported 33
　socioeconomic 51, 52
　sources 28
decisional balance 61
Dela*WELL* 39, 57, 74
Dela*WELL* University 165-166, 167
demonstrations 11, 12, 47, 48
Department of Health and Human Services (HHS) 51
DermaScan 46
dietitians 10
DiPasquale, Ray 46
discretionary time 8, 58, 59
displays 12, 48, 53
dramatic relief 61
Drink Up 112, 113

E

ecological models 76
Edington, Dee, Dr. 26
education programs 18
　community-based 78
　formats of 36-37, 39
education sector 6. *See also* schools
educational materials 12, 39
educational workshops 8, 39
elected officials 8
employees. *See also* worksites
　absenteeism 28
　engaging 57
　government 7, 19, 39, 46, 57
　job satisfaction 8, 28
　participation 9
　productivity 28
　recognition 20, 73
　self-leadership 27
　surveying 28
employment 5
engagement
　and enjoyment 45, 53
　and environment 45
　knowing needs and wants 28
　senior-level 26
　sustaining 45
　and timing 53
environment. *See also* organizational culture

adapting 45
advocating change 10
safety 44, 45
supports 76
environmental reevaluation 61
evaluation 18, 71
Evans, Adrienne 51
event planning 10
evidence-based practice 16, 18, 22, 50, 52
exercise. *See* physical activity
exercise instruction 45
expertise 10
extrinsic rewards 62

F

faith-based organizations 6, 9
families
　behavioral influence 76
　opportunities for 10
　support from 64
　time with 58
Farmers Markets 109
Farrell, Stephen 7
fast food 49
fitness 6
Fitness Bee 102-103
Fitting in Fitness 91-92
Fitzgerald, Rick 25
foods
　in cafeterias 77
　from farmers markets 77
　in schools 78
food samples 48
food stamps 77
foundations 70-71
Framingham Heart Study 63
free samples 48
fun 45, 53

G

Gainesville, Florida 16
Gainesville Health and Fitness Club 16
Genetic Information Non-Discrimination Act (GINA) 32, 40
Get Fit, Rhode Island! 7, 19
Gifford, David, Dr. 7
global health care crisis 4
Glo Germ 11
goals
　personal 63, 64
　of programs 16
　setting 34-35
　SMART 34-35
Goetzel, Ron 17, 45
Good for You 45
Good to Great (Collins) 72
government programs 5
government regulations 40

Great American Smokeout 55
groups
　accommodating 10
　discounts for 5

H

hands-on demonstrations 48
health
　determinants of 75
　expenditures 4
　indicators 74
　of minority populations 52
　promotion 17
Health and Productivity Management (HPM) 17
health assessments. *See* health risk questionnaire (HRQ)
health care
　costs 4, 7, 16, 59
　coverage 4
　global crisis 4, 59
health clubs 12, 38, 57, 58
health disparities 51
health education 10
Health Enhancement Research Organization (HERO) 78
health fairs 46
health insurance
　copayments 8
　providers 31
Health Insurance Portability and Accountability Act (HIPAA) 32, 40
health interest surveys 28
　versus risk surveys 31
　sample 29-30
health professionals. *See* wellness professionals
health risk assessment 32
health risk questionnaire (HRQ) 19
　administering 32-33
　completion rate by incentive value and commitment level 67*f*
　confidentiality 32
　online assessment 32
　paper assessment 32
　reliability 31
　sample questions 32
　sources for 31
　validation 31
healthcare sector 6
health screenings 33, 58
Healthier US Schools Challenge Program 11
Healthy America initiative 5, 6
Healthy Book Club 164
Healthy Eating Every Day 121
Healthy Meetings 116-117
Healthy People 2010 51

Healthy States Summit 6
heart disease 39
helping relationship 62
HERO. *See* Health Enhancement
    Research Organization
    (HERO)
Hewitt Associates 37, 54, 59
hospitals 6
HRQ. *See* health risk questionnaire
    (HRQ)
Huckabee, Mike, Governor 5
Human Kinetics 52
A Hydration Challenge 112, 113

I

incentives 8
    and financial outcomes 8
    for health risk questionnaires 33
    and HRQ completion rate 67*f*
    immediacy 33, 68
    promotional items as 67-68
    to reinforce healthy culture 27
    role of 65-66
    suggested ideas 67
    for wellness champions 20
industry sector 6
infrastructure 18, 71
interest surveys 28, 29-30, 31
International Health, Racquet
        and Sportsclub Association
        (IHRSA) 59
intervention programs 18, 37, 39
intrinsic motivation 60, 62, 65

J

job satisfaction 8, 28
Join the Club 101
Journal of Occupational and Envi-
        ronmental Medicine 17
Just Move It 39, 97-99

K

Kapetanios, Jean 36
Katz, David, MD, MPH 49, 90
Kick Colds and Flu 11, 132-133
kiosks 32, 78
Know Your Health 157-158
Know Your Numbers 148-149
Kotler, Philip 49
Kumar, Rajiv 55

L

Lactation Support 151-152
Laugh It Up! 125
leadership
    effective actions of 20
    engagement 73
    inspiration from 20
    meetings 20
    operational 26
    participation in programs 20
    roles of 73

in schools 20
senior-level support 19-20,
    73-74
support 4, 9, 73
and vision 26
learning theory 62
Lee, Debbie 16
legal issues 40
leisure time 8, 58, 59, 65
lessons learned 18, 42
Let's Dance 9, 104
Let's Move campaign 6, 11
lifestyles
    awareness 36
    individual commitment to 27
    physically active 6
    risky behaviors 36
    sedentary 75
locations 57, 58
logos 47
Lunch and Learn 110-111

M

Make It Stick 144-145
management. *See* leadership
marketing. *See* social marketing
martial arts 10
Maslow, Abraham 60
mass media 6
massage 10, 48
mastering experience 63
measurement 17, 18, 28. *See*
        also data
    of goals 34
    of outcomes 42
    process 40, 42
    qualitative 40
    quantitative 40
media sector 6
medical insurance claims 28, 74
medical screening 40
meetings
    with decision makers 21
    productivity 25
    walking 4
    of wellness champions 25
mental health 32
Meyers, David, Dr. 76
Michelin Tires 54
minority groups 52
monitoring 18, 40
motivation 62, 64, 65
Moving Meetings 96
municipalities 6, 9
Musical Happy Hour 130
My Physical Activity Tracker 99
My Pledge 159-160

N

Nashville's Metro Parks and Rec-
        reation Department 9

National Business Group on Health
    (NBGH) 78
National Governors Association
    (NGA) 5, 6
National Physical Activity Plan
    (NPAP) 6, 7
NGA. *See* National Governors
    Association (NGA)
non-profit organizations 6
NPAP. *See* National Physical Activ-
    ity Plan (NPAP)
nurses 10
nutrition
    classes 10, 40
    poor 11, 75
    in schools 11
    specialist in 10
Nutrition Detectives 12, 106-107

O

Obama, Michelle, First Lady 6, 11
obesity 4, 11, 49
Observe Health 150
online programs 53, 66
on-site services 5
operations leadership 26
organizational culture 16, 26
    engaging 45
    enjoyment 4, 45
    evaluating 27
    five pillars 26-27
    reinforcing 27
    and verbal communication 27
    and vision 26
    visual signs of 27
organizations. *See also* communi-
        cation; worksites
    benefits of worksite wellness 8
    commitment 17
    current climate 17
    health indicators 74-75
    individuals' sense of value to 75
    infrastructure 19
    wellness goals 16-17
outcome evaluations 72
outdoor meetings 4

P

parks and recreation 5, 6
participation waivers 40
partnerships 6, 7, 10
PawSox and Prostrates 135-136
peer networks 9
performance measures 17
Pet Therapy 131
pharmaceutical claims 28
physical activity
    adherence to 8
    barriers to 8, 64
    enjoyment 64
    national plan for 6

and self-motivation 64
tracking 99
Physical Activity Tracker 99
Pickering, David 59
Pink Spirit Week 140
Play Ball 95
policy 10, 76-77
Porras 22, 74
Portion Distortion 108
PowerPoint presentations 51
prevention 4, 17, 32
price 57-58
privacy 32, 40, 58
process of change 61-62
Pro-Change 141
Prochaska, J., Dr. 59, 60
product
    delivery timing 52-53
    need for 52
    program content 52
    target population 51-52
professionals. *See* wellness professionals
Program Satisfaction survey 41
program support 9
programs
    cost 64
    quality 64
    types 8-9
Project Active 52
promotional materials 39
public health sector 6
public opinion 8
public policy 76
public-private partnerships 6, 7

Q

quality assurance 27
quality of life 4, 17
questionnaires. *See* health risk questionnaire (HRQ)

R

Raytheon Healthy Worksite Award 153
recognition
    of champions 20, 73
    of employees 20, 73
    of participants 20
reinforcement management 62
relationship building 23, 24
reporting 17, 18, 42
research 18
resources
    allocation of 73
    budgets 36, 39, 58
    in communities 10
    for execution of NPAP 7
    online 28, 78, 79
    organizational 17
return on investment (ROI)

measuring 28
studies 17
of traditional *versus* comprehensive programming 18
of wellness programs 8
rewards 62. *See also* incentives
Rhode Island
    Cancer Prevention Research Center 59
    Dept. of Labor and Training 25
    Get Fit program 6, 7, 19
risk assessment. *See* Health Risk Questionnaire (HRQ)

S

safety
    environment 44, 45
    in schools 79
Salo, LLC 4
Samuelson, Michael 7
satisfaction surveys 28, 40, 41
school districts 5, 11
School Health Index (SHI) 79, 142-143
schools
    academic success and health 11
    curriculum integration 12
    demands on time 11
    environmental approach 78
    food menus 78
    hand-washing campaign 11
    leadership support 20
    physical education in 11
    policies 77
    staff programs 12
    wellness committees 11
    wellness strategies 12
Schrader, Aaron, MS 74, 75
scorecard 78
Screen Savers 168
seasonal offerings 10, 40
sedentary lifestyles 75
self-directed programs 8
self-efficacy 9, 61
self-efficacy theory 62-63
self-liberation 61
self-motivation 64
self-reevaluation 61
Seminar Registration Form 167
senior centers 9
senior leadership. *See* leadership
Shape Up, RI 55
Shape Up the Nation 63, 93-94
short-duration programs 8, 11
SMART goals 34-35
smoking 34, 38, 75
smoking ban 76
social cognitive theory 63
social-ecological model 76*f*
social liberation 61

social marketing 49-50. *See also* wellness promotion
    definition of 49
    demographics 51
    four P's 50-51
    program delivery 51-53
    socioeconomic data 51, 52
    strategies 36
    target audience 50, 51-52
social networks 9, 63-64, 75
social opportunities 10
social support
    and behavior change 63
    and exercise adherence 8
    and self-efficacy 63
socioeconomic factors 75
SparkPeople 100
specialists 10
spokespersons 55
sports 6, 10
staging 45-46
    demonstrations 47, 48
    by engaging the senses 47-48
    plan preparation 48
    product samples 48
    between programs 48
StairWELL to Better Health 86-87
state employees 7, 19, 39, 46, 57
state health departments 31
steering committees 19, 26
stimulus control 62
Stop, Stretch, and Breathe 126-127
strategic plan 35-36
strategic thinking 22
stress 8, 32, 40
Stress-Less Day 53, 128-129
stress management 39, 40, 51
stress surveys 28
substance use 11
success 18, 72
Sun Smarts 137
Survey Monkey 28
surveys
    customizing 28
    health interest 29-30
    job satisfaction 28
    program satisfaction 41

T

Taitel, Michael 66
Take the Stairs 38
taxes 77
teams
    bonding 25
    building 22
    champions 17
    competitions 55
    interdisciplinary 17
    key members 17
themes 48

Third Annual Obesity Congress 49
tobacco use 34, 38, 75
trademarks 56
traditional programming 18
trans fat 77
transportation
    by bicycle 77
    pedestrian walkways 78
    sector 6
    walk-to-school policy 77
transtheoretical model (TTM)
    60-62
treadmill workstations 4. *See*
    also Moving Meetings
TrestleTree Health Coaching 169

U

UnitedHealthcare of New England
    7, 36, 46
University of Michigan 31
University of Rhode Island 7
    Cancer Prevention Research
        Center 61
urban design 6
U.S. Centers for Disease Control
    and Prevention (CDC) 50,
    52, 76, 79
U.S. Department of Health and
    Human Services (HHS) 51

V

"value meals" 49
Veggin' Out 122
Vélib' 77
vending machines 76, 77
vendors 5, 46, 48
vicarious experience 63
Virtual Reminders 161
vision 35
    communicating 73
    creation 26
visual aids 47
visual communication 27, 31,
    38, 47
visual learning 47
Vitality 162-163
volunteer organizations 6

W

waivers 40
walking meetings 4
walking paths 76, 78
weight loss 34, 49
WELCOA. *See* Wellness Council
    of America (WELCOA)
wellness champions 19, 20, 23
    appointment of 20, 23
    as cheerleaders 24
    incentives for 20
    meetings 25

recognition of 20, 24-25
relationship building 24
selection 24
team bonding 25
workload 24
Wellness Council of America
    (WELCOA) 7, 16, 18, 28, 79
    strategic plan components
        35-36
wellness director 19, 21
    commitment 22-23
    enthusiasm 21, 22
    essential qualities of 22-23
    experience of 22
    meeting with decision makers
        21
    planning roles 20
    selection qualities 22-23
    support of leadership 20
Wellness Impact Scorecard 154
wellness initiatives
    beginning 16
    collaboration 6, 7, 21
    focusing 34
    implementation timeline 35
    launch strategies 18
    "lone ranger" approach 23
    multidisciplinary representa-
        tion 24
    phased launches 17
    proposals 21
    public kick-offs 20
    sense of ownership 24
    steps to building 18
    successful themes 17
    tailoring to population 75
    timing 17, 18, 52-53
    written plan 35-36
wellness professionals
    client base 5
    leveraging health crisis 4
    revenue building 5
    service offerings 5
wellness programs. *See also* well-
    ness initiatives; wellness
    strategies
    awareness 18, 38
    community offerings 5
    convenience of 8, 57
    costs 57-59
    cultivating 42
    demand for 4-5
    determining effectiveness 17
    educational 18, 39
    for government employees 4-5
    in-house 5
    for intervention 39
    prioritizing 20
    selection considerations 39-40

settings for 12, 57, 58
state-level 5-6
time commitment 54
visibility 58
wellness promotion
    announcements 23, 54
    bulletin boards 48, 78
    delivery methods 55
    displays 12, 48, 53
    educational programs 39
    enthusiasm 57
    materials 12, 39
    range of venues 6
    repetition 56
    sales tips 57
    signage 56
    spokesperson for 55
    strategy variety 53
    tips 56
    touch points 56
wellness strategies 37-38
    in communities 10, 77, 78
    for schools 12, 77, 78
    for worksites 8-9, 77, 78
Weygand, Robert 7
WIIFM: What's in It For Me? 118
workday programs 8
workers' compensation 28, 74
work–life balance 75
workshops 8, 39
Worksite Health Promotion
    (Chenoweth) 18
worksites. *See also* organizations
    cafeterias 77
    employee participation 9
    employer-employee relations 77
    environment 77-78
    morale 8
    on-the-job recognition 75
    policies 77
    program strategies 8-9
    program timing 9
    social interaction in 75
    stress 8, 75
    support 9
    workweek hours 7, 8
Worksite Wellness Council of
    Rhode Island (WWCRI) 7
World Health Organization 49

Y

Yale-Griffin Prevention Research
    Center 49, 90
YMCA 45
YMCA's Healthy Family Home
    146-147

Z

Zaltman, Gerald 49
Zero Trends (Edington) 26